PENGUIN BOOKS

WE ARE ALL THE SAME

Jim Wooten is the senior correspondent for ABC News's *Nightline*. He has served as a bureau chief, national correspondent, and White House correspondent for *The New York Times*. He is the recipient of the 2002 John Chancellor Award for Excellence in Journalism. He and his wife, Patience O'Connor, live in Washington, D.C. They have five daughters and six grandchildren.

Praise for *We Are All the Same*

"This is a lyrical, beautiful book about life and death. As a story of friendship as unlikely as it is wonderful, it reminds me of nothing so much as *Tuesdays with Morrie*."
—David Halberstam

"Wooten has pulled off something close to miraculous with Nkosi Johnson's story. He has taken off the rubber gloves, torn away the plastic mask and touched the face of HIV/AIDS with compassion and humanity. Instead of mind-numbing statistics and arm's-length reporting, Wooten gives us the very flesh-and-blood 'not an angel' Nkosi; his young, dying, biological mother, Daphne Khumalo; his remarkable adoptive mother, Gail Johnson; and his best friend, Eric Nichols. The characters tumble off the pages of this remarkable, short book in full cry. Wooten has a gift of the quick draw, and we are quickly drawn into the story. Simply put, it's difficult to look away."
—Alexandra Fuller, *Chicago Tribune*

"Amazing and tender. . . . Everyone knows Wooten is possibly the best storyteller on TV, and in this special book he brings home the tragedy of AIDS and the fact of a friendship that went deep."
—Liz Smith, *New York Post*

"Wooten has been able to craft a remarkable tale of the disease by chronicling the story of one little black South African boy named Nkosi Johnson in *We Are All the Same*, a book that comes across as painful and tragic on one hand and hopeful and joyous on the other. . . . The story Wooten describes, if written as fiction, would probably come off as trite and sentimental. As reality, it remains a striking reminder of how disastrous this disease has been for southern Africa, especially considering the progress that could have been made post-apartheid."

—*Los Angeles Times*

"Jim Wooten has long been the best storyteller on television. His reporting about Nkosi Johnson has been heart-rending, compassionate and tender. Now with this very special book, he brings the tragedy of AIDS to unforgettable life through the story of this remarkable and loving circle of caregivers. If you can read about Jim laying his white-haired, six-foot-two frame down on a bed to say a final goodbye to this twelve-year-old without tears, you have no heart."

—Benjamin Bradlee, author of *A Good Life*

"Jim Wooten has written a beautiful and terrifying love story about the magnificence of a dying child, the gifts he gave, the inspiration he spread, and the stubborn and lethal ignorance of the government that should have loved him."

—Roger Wilkins, author of *Jefferson's Pillow: The Founding Fathers and the Dilemma of Black Patriotism*

"A touching love story between a young Zulu boy born with AIDS and his adoptive mother, a white South African woman who has made AIDS activism into her life's mission."

—*Reader's Digest* (Editor's Choice)

"The moving life story of Xolani Nkosi Johnson, a Zulu South African born HIV-positive during the last year of apartheid. . . . Wooten rightly disregards journalistic distance and writes himself into the work, making it read like a contemplative literary memoir, with just enough of the country's history, culture, politics—and grim mortality rates—to give their story context."

—*TimeOut New York*

"The issue of AIDS in Africa . . . becomes powerfully real in *We Are All the Same*, a slender volume that conveys the depth and breadth of the unfolding tragedy . . . in clear-eyed prose. . . . By telling Nkosi's story, Wooten illuminates the story in a way that the grim numbers cannot. He has written that rarest of things: a book that has the power to change lives."
        —*OregonLive*

"Jim Wooten, an award-winning senior correspondent for ABC News, has written a book to break our hearts. But it is also a call to action . . . The more Jim Wootens there are to bring us the AIDS story straight, the better the chances that Nkosi's fight goes on."
        —*Houston Chronicle*

"*We Are All the Same* is a small book costing a mere $20. Most of the profits go to AIDS orphans in Africa. This won't make Jim Wooten rich. Nkosi Johnson already did that. His incredible story will make you richer too."
        —*The Huntsville Times*

"A veteran TV newsman's heartfelt account of the relationship between Nkosi, a Zulu boy with AIDS, and Gail Johnson, his white South African foster mother, a woman committed to giving her doomed, beloved child the best life possible. . . . Woven into this love story between a black child and his white foster mother is the bleak tale of South Africa's failure to deal with the massive problem of AIDS. . . . The story of one valiant little boy and his remarkable foster mother goes right to the heart."
        —*Kirkus Reviews* (starred review)

"An extraordinarily moving account of a courageous South African boy's battle with AIDS. . . . This powerful account puts a human face on a catastrophic epidemic that grows worse daily."
        — *PublishersWeekly* (starred review)

WE ARE ALL
THE SAME

A Story of a Boy's Courage

and a Mother's Love

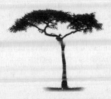

JIM WOOTEN

PENGUIN BOOKS

To Clara, my mother

PENGUIN BOOKS

Published by the Penguin Group
Penguin Group (USA) Inc., 375 Hudson Street, New York, New York 10014, U.S.A.
Penguin Group (Canada), 10 Alcorn Avenue, Toronto,
Ontario, Canada M4V 3B2 (a division of Pearson Penguin Canada Inc.)
Penguin Books Ltd, 80 Strand, London WC2R 0RL, England
Penguin Ireland, 25 St Stephen's Green, Dublin 2, Ireland (a division of Penguin Books Ltd)
Penguin Group (Australia), 250 Camberwell Road, Camberwell,
Victoria 3124, Australia (a division of Pearson Australia Group Pty Ltd)
Penguin Books India Pvt Ltd, 11 Community Centre,
Panchsheel Park, New Delhi – 110 017, India
Penguin Group (NZ), cnr Airborne and Rosedale Roads, Albany,
Auckland 1310, New Zealand (a division of Pearson New Zealand Ltd)
Penguin Books (South Africa) (Pty) Ltd, 24 Sturdee Avenue,
Rosebank, Johannesburg 2196, South Africa

Penguin Books Ltd, Registered Offices:
80 Strand, London WC2R 0RL, England

First published in the United States of America by The Penguin Press,
a member of Penguin Group (USA) Inc. 2004
Published in Penguin Books 2005

1   3   5   7   9   10   8   6   4   2

THE LIBRARY OF CONGRESS HAS CATALOGED
THE HARDCOVER EDITION AS FOLLOWS:
Wooten, Jim.
We are all the same : a story of a boy's courage and a mother's love / Jim Wooten.
p.   cm.
ISBN 1-59420-028-9 (hc.)
ISBN 0 14 30.3599 1 (pbk.)
1. Johnson, Nkosi 1989–2001—Health.   2. AIDS (Disease) in children—
Patients—South Africa—Biography.   I. Title.
RJ387.A25 W66 2004
362.196'9792'0083—dc22
[B]   2004049526

Printed in the United States of America

INTRODUCTION

The secret of journalism is that its practitioners are paid to live lives of sweet expectation. Even the most indolent members of our tribe come to understand that on any given day, sheer amazement could well be waiting. In fact, over the years of my career, I have always been astonished *not* to be astonished. Still, when I first landed in Africa a long time ago, I was unprepared for its impact on me. Even in that initial exposure, brief as it was, I discovered such beauty, such vast vistas of nature and culture and history, reaching far beyond my own culture's ordinary measurements of such things.

So I returned to Africa again and again, not merely for the place itself but for the people I met and the rich stories they shared with me. I heard the words "Mother Africa" said in many languages and dialects, and over the years I came to say those words, in English, more and more myself. It is an appropriate name for every one of us to use, of course. Beyond any symbolism, it really *is* mother to us all—a life cradle from which we all have come and in which we all have roots, whatever the color of our skin. I recall mentioning the power of this connection to Richard Leakey over dinner one evening in Nairobi. The renowned anthropologist, a white man who considered himself to be as much a Kenyan as Jomo Kenyatta was, smiled and said, "Africa, old chap, is everybody's home." Perhaps that notion is part of what kept taking me back, the sense that in some odd way I actually was going home.

No doubt, too, that as a reporter I was drawn by the number of important stories Africa presented to me and by the memories those stories left me, both horrible and beautiful: that nightmarish moment in Congo when I watched a Rwandan mother toss her baby, dead of typhus, onto a mounting pile of bodies, then turn and walk calmly down a dusty road toward the distant mountains; that hair-raising afternoon in Zimbabwe when the small plane in which I was a passenger crashed into a field infested with spitting cobras; that time in Ethiopia when I was gloriously pummeled and pushed to the ground by dozens of laughing kids who had never before seen a white man; that long day I spent with Nelson Mandela's wife and grandson while he was still in prison.

This book began as one of those stories.

It is about the relationship between a black child who never grew up and a white woman who never gave up. It has neither a happy ending nor even a promising beginning, for the child had no choice and no chance, and the woman knew all along what she was up against. Had they lived their lives separate from one another, they might have become more or less ordinary people. Not that they would have been unimportant, but, alone and apart, each might have gone unnoticed and unremembered in the larger flow of African life. Together, however, their impact was considerable.

My own role in their story is minimal. I'm an aging if not yet ancient reporter and should have known better, but even though I made an honest effort to keep a journalist's discreet distance, to remain emotionally uninvolved in what was seen and heard, I was powerfully drawn to this child and this woman, as much as I have been drawn to Africa itself. Almost before I understood what was happening, we became friends.

So, with some reluctance and not much practice, I have inserted myself into certain aspects of their story, only to provide background and context—and also, I suppose, to reinforce its pull, even on someone quite determined to remain detached. It was my intention when I began writing their story to maintain a steady and straightforward narrative; eventually, however, I found that a few small circles and digressions were unavoidable. Perhaps there are too many, but it is difficult if not impossible to grasp a story like this one—a story that, as will become clear, carries so much historical, emotional, and political weight—without also coming to grips with the historical, emotional, political terrain on which it occurred.

I also realize that, like most really good stories, this one is bound to be diminished simply by the telling. My reporting cannot reconstruct the reality, nor can my writing capture the richness and power of their lives. Still, it's my belief that anyone who has the good fortune to cross paths with people as exceptional as this child and this woman is obligated to pass along their story, no matter how flawed the medium or faulty the method.

It is with that sense of inherent imperfection that I have tried to do just that. I am simply passing it along in these pages, in the sure and certain knowledge that it is really quite beyond me.

WE ARE ALL THE SAME

PROLOGUE

On my way into the house from the car, I heard a child's voice from the other side of a thick hedge running along the driveway. I thought this was probably the kid—and although it's never been my habit to eavesdrop, I had, after all, traveled several thousand miles, all the way to the bottom of Africa, specifically to see him, to broadcast his story on an American television network. So it was no great ethical stretch for me to rationalize a small moment of eavesdropping. It seemed not so much an invasion of his privacy as an innocent opportunity to size him up before we sat down together later that afternoon for an on-camera interview.

I peeked through the bushes and saw a little boy pacing back and forth in a scruffy garden beside the shabby house.

We are all the same, he was saying.

He paused and repeated the phrase.

We are all the same.

I was sure he couldn't see me, and he was certain he was alone, talking only to himself.

We are not different from one another, he continued.

Once again he paused, apparently stumped. He glanced down at the paper in his hand, then looked up and out into the distance before adding a few forgotten words to those he had remembered.

We are all the same.

We are not different from one another.

We all belong to one family.

He nodded, pleased with himself.

His thin voice perfectly matched his frail physique, and the clothing he wore seemed to diminish him even further: a bulky sweater much too large, cargo pants dragging the ground around his sneakers, and a baseball cap settled down around his ears, its Chicago Bulls logo nearly the size of his face. A stiff breeze would have blown him away, and I thought he could not possibly have been eleven years old, the age listed for him in the sheaf of research I'd read on the plane. He looked no more than six or seven—and yet there he was rehearsing a speech I'd been told he would soon be making to an in-person audience of several thousand people, as well as to millions watching on satellite television. Of course, it was possible that he was *not* the right kid, not the one I'd come to Johannesburg to see. Either that or he was a midget. I made a mental note to check and confirm his age.

We are all the same, he was saying again.

We are not different from one another.

We all belong to one family.

As I would learn, these were not idle words for him, nor merely rhetorical themes for his speech. His constant mantra was *equality,* his passionate gospel *family,* a concept with which he was thoroughly familiar, since he had several of them. There was the one into which he had been born but from which he had been separated and to some degree alienated for several years; there was another within which he lived his day-to-day life; and, of course, there was the family in which his membership was entirely involuntary but which he had embraced nevertheless.

We are all the same.

We are not different from one another.

We all belong to one family.

Between each phrase and the next, he paused and grinned—his white teeth sparkling against the dark skin of his face —and I realized he was playing to several cameras he pretended were in the garden, shamelessly hamming it up, conjuring for the purposes of his rehearsal the real ones he'd been told would be rolling when he actually took the stage.

We are all the same.

Smile.

We are not different from one another.

Smile.

We all belong to one family.

Smile.

In America this kid could run for Congress.

I liked him anyway—or at any rate I found myself immediately impressed with his patience and his determination. He seemed more than willing to practice his lines until he had mastered them, no matter how much time that might require. There was also about him a certain guileless charm—even in those first few moments I was captivated by his unassuming innocence. The space usually maintained between me and the people in my stories was rapidly shrinking, and I knew I was granting myself an indulgence for the worst possible reason—because . . . well, because the kid was cute.

We are all the same.
We are not different from one another.
We all belong to one family.

It suddenly struck me that his words were ringing a distant bell—

We are all the same.

—like some old song long hidden away—

We are not different from one another.

—on some dark ledge of my brain—

We all belong to one family.

—until, at last, it came to me.

We love and we laugh, we hurt and we cry, we live and we die.

Yes, of course. In his soft, singsong soprano, he was recit-
ing an adaptation—*his* adaptation, as it turned out—of Shake-
speare's best lines in *The Merchant of Venice,* those memorable
words spoken by Shylock in behalf of his maligned and mar
ginalized tribe:

> *I am a Jew.*
> *Hath not a Jew eyes?*
> *Hath not a Jew hands, organs, dimensions, senses, affections,*
> *   passions? . . .*
> *If you prick us, do we not bleed?*
> *If you tickle us, do we not laugh?*
> *If you poison us, do we not die?*

The kid was speaking not for the Jews, of course, but
rather for that exponentially expanding family he had not
asked to join but of which he was nevertheless a part: the millions of Africans who carried a deadly virus in their bodies, an
infection that had not only doomed them but damned them as
well, had made of them social pariahs, punished by their countries and cultures and communities simply because they were
ill, stigmatized as the new lepers of the new millennium.

The kid was speaking for them—

We are all the same.

—and for himself—

We are all the same.

—and, in a way, for all the maligned and marginalized of
the earth.

> *We are not different from one another.*
> *We all belong to one family.*
> *We love and we laugh.*
> *We hurt and we cry.*
> *We live and we die.*

He seemed not quite pleased with his recitation of the last
line and tried it with a different emphasis and body language.

> *We live . . .*

He paused and grinned, slightly opened his arms, the palms
of his hands turned upward, and shrugged his narrow shoulders, as though he did not care about his final words.

> *. . . and we die.*

I retreated into the house, confident that he had not been
aware of my presence and stunned by the impact he'd managed
to make on me in just those few brief moments. I had more
than enough questions for three or four interviews, for five
or six stories—questions like, who was this kid, and where
did he come from, and where did he get so much grit and
chutzpah, and how smart was he, and what made him tick, and
what made him different, and how genuine was his supposed

indifference to death, and what would happen to him, and, in the end, who the hell would care?

That was the beginning, that brisk afternoon in the South African spring of 2000. Over and over the next year or so, I would seek and find the answers to a few, if not all, of those questions—and although there was no way I could have known that day, of course, just how personally rewarding the process would be, as I explored the labyrinth of his history and sifted through the artifacts of his life, I would also unearth a treasure that would enrich my own life forever.

Little by little, I would discover Nkosi.

ONE

He was born in a place that did not exist.

By 1989 the name and the boundaries of Zululand had all but vanished from the maps of South Africa, its vast territory attached to provinces with less-exotic names, its best acreage confiscated and given to others, its people scattered about the country in ugly ghettos or squatters' camps. Yet its hardiest memories had survived among many of the elderly who had once lived there, and to this day its more powerful myths persist among their children and their children's children as well.

And no wonder.

Zululand had been a truly memorable place, occupying as much as a quarter of what would eventually become South Africa, stretching from the beaches of the Indian Ocean to a rugged mountain range called u Khahlanha, "the Barrier of

Spears." In some parts it had blossomed with acacia trees and aloes, in others with sugarcane and citrus groves thick with oranges and lemons. It had not only the world's second-highest waterfall but also the wondrous Valley of a Thousand Hills, which had been created, said the Zulus, when God crumpled the world in his hands just at the point of discarding it in disgust . . . before deciding against it—and over the years, even into its declining days, it had remained a haunting source and setting for the storytellers of the country.

In the opening pages of *Cry, the Beloved Country,* the poignant novel about a disintegrating Zulu family, Alan Paton depicted the barren land left to the tribe by the late 1940s and, with bitter brevity, described what had befallen the people struggling to survive on it.

"The streams are all dry," he wrote.

Too many cattle feed upon the grass and too many fires have burned it. Stand shod upon it for it is coarse and sharp and the stones cut under the feet. It is not kept or guarded or cared for. It no longer keeps men, guards men, cares for men.

The great red hills stand desolate and the earth has torn away like flesh. The lightning flashes over them, the clouds pour down upon them, the dead streams come to life, full of the red blood of the earth. Down in the valleys, women scratch the soil that is left and the maize hardly reaches the height of a man. They are valleys of old men and old women, of mothers and children. The men are away. The soil cannot keep them anymore.

Paton christened his fictional family Kumalo, a common enough name among Zulus, roughly the equivalent of Smith or Jones in America. For long generations, reaching far back into the previous century, tens of thousands of flesh-and-blood Zulu families had borne it, including the one from which the boy would come. His maternal grandmother was Ruth Khumalo, and as her name would inextricably connect her to the roots of her tribe, her life would mirror its descent into the madness of postwar South Africa. She would spend years in what was left of Zululand, but she never knew what it once had been, had never stood atop one of those thousand hills to gaze out on high grasslands so perfect for livestock and farming, had never seen for herself—as millions of white tourists have seen—the Tulego River's breathtaking cascade. None of that would ever be a part of her life, for Ruth Khumalo would experience Zululand only in the grim terms of Alan Paton's fictional vision.

Ruth Khumalo was born in 1950 into that first misbegotten generation of black South Africans who would live under the official strictures of apartheid, a Kafkaesque universe of repressive racial regulations that had begun to take malevolent shape in 1948 when Afrikaners—mainly of Dutch and French descent—won control of the South African government from the British and immediately set about reinforcing the dominance of whites in the country. In Afrikaans—their language—*apartheid* simply means "apartness," a benign and harmless concept, but as it came to be applied to black South Africans, it translated into a brutal system of segregation and subjugation that would last for nearly half a century and eventually subject the country to international condemnation, to economic and political pressures that would finally contribute to its demise.

Although "apartheid" is now a familiar term in much of the world, a few brief details of its history seem necessary to explain its grotesque impact on the life of Ruth Khumalo as well as on her children and their children, including the boy. Its evil evolution began with the forced registration-by-race of everyone in the country, soon followed by the division of every town and city into areas in which only those of a particular race could legally reside. Few whites were affected, but hundreds of thousands of black citizens were rousted from their homes and neighborhoods and forced to live only in segregated townships near the urban centers.

Next, so-called pass laws severely restricted the movement of black South Africans around their own country—and although none of these measures represented a dramatic departure from the de facto customs and traditions to which South Africa had long been accustomed, the Afrikaners laid them on in increasingly minute detail, codified them, hardened them into legislation and then law. Having dealt with the cities and towns, they launched a massive rural land grab, evicting millions of black South Africans from the fields and pastures on which they had lived for generations and offering in exchange enclaves carved from the least-fertile acreage in the country. Ostensibly tribal, these Bantustans were devised not only to open up more good land for white farmers but also to make it appear—to outsiders, at least—that whites were merely one of many African tribes happily living together while separately sharing the land. In reality the goal was to jam more than half the national population into about 10 percent of the land, to make 40 million people more or less disappear. The Bantustans were nothing more than wilderness ghettos, where even subsistence survival was next to impossible.

Ruth Khumalo was born on one of them.

Years later she would tell her own children that among the first phrases she learned to say was *Kodwa silambile*. In the Zulu language, it means, "We are hungry." She also learned, of course, that the word *Zulu* itself means "paradise." She would never understand why.

Like thousands of desperate black families, hers simply walked away from the Bantustan, looking for some improvement in their lives. Many headed for the already overflowing townships established near the all-white cities. By the mid-1950s, in fact, the townships were home to a majority of the country's black population, but they were such rough and rowdy places that many of the rural dispossessed chose not to join the urban rush—too weak or too poor, too unskilled and too uneducated, too tired and too frightened to be comfortable in them. Besides, their pastoral legacy was strong. They had lived all their days in the countryside, and it was there that many of them chose to remain.

Yet once they chose to leave the Bantustans, they had no choice but to become rootless nomads, wandering the rural reaches in search of someplace—anyplace—to settle, legally or otherwise. For Ruth Khumalo and her children and their children, this was among the most damning legacies of apartheid. In the land of their birth, they and millions like them

were homeless, with no more status than illegal aliens. Zululand was no longer theirs. It had been stolen.

For a tribe that had occupied such a vast swath of southern Africa, it had been a precipitous decline. For much of the
nineteenth century, the Zulus had been the continent's ar-
chetypal warriors, famous for inventing new weapons and
adopting innovative battlefield tactics. Their fierce warriors
had followed a succession of bold chiefs, most notably the
shrewd Shaka, who led them first against their black neighbors
and then against waves of white Europeans. Even though the
whites were prone to turn on each other, their internecine
squabbles proved irrelevant. In the end the Zulus—like most
other African tribes faced with European colonization—were
vanquished.

In such a long and bloody process, Zululand became a
mother lode of legend. The last of the Bonaparte line, the son
of Napolean III, was slain there, by Zulus. Not far from where
he fell, more than a thousand British soldiers were slaughtered
in one day, by Zulus. In another battle, white settlers killed so
many Zulus that a nearby stream was renamed Blood River.
A youthful Winston Churchill, working as a reporter, was captured in the same war in which a young Mohandas Gandhi was
serving as a volunteer medic. The Englishman escaped, the Indian survived, and each went home to other matters, but history was not nearly so kind to the Zulus. By the end of the
nineteenth century, most of the land they had conquered and
captured over the years was all gone.

Still, even that did not seem to change who they were, or at
least who they tried to be. Squeezed into a shrunken fraction

of the space they had formerly occupied, the Zulus nevertheless maintained many of the traditions that had become inherent parts of their culture. Paramount among these was the
singular importance of the family. It was, in fact, the bedrock
of their character and their community, the overarching value
of the tribe. In every Zulu village, the aged were respected and
revered, the disabled and the orphans embraced and cared for,
the children treasured and taught. While polygamy was customary, husbands protected and provided for their wives no
matter how many they had. The women, in turn, honored their
men. Marriages were sacred and enduring, families stable and
strong.

Then, in the early twentieth century, British colonial authorities imposed a tax on the Zulus that had to be paid in
cash. Those who did not pay it were subject to fines or impris-
onment or both, but while most Zulus were willing to pay it,
few had any cash. The basis of their economy was livestock, its
primary currency cattle.

Almost immediately—by the hundreds at first, then by the
thousands—the men left their villages to find jobs in a bur-
geoning industrial economy where they could earn the cash to
pay the tax that would at least keep them legal. Only a tiny
fraction of their wives and children accompanied them in a
massive male exodus from the countryside, just as the British
had planned all along. The tax created a cheap labor force for
the whites who owned the coal mines and the diamond mines
and the mills. In a generation or two, the Zulus were farmers
and herders no more, no longer proudly self-sufficient, and

their families, once the very soul of their tribe, quickly began to crumble. For a brief moment, they rose en masse in a bloody insurrection, a fierce tax rebellion doomed from the start and quickly extinguished by the British, who had not only the reins of government in their hands but most of the guns as well.

Four generations later the boy was born, in a land that no longer existed, in a village with no name. It is still there, somewhere out in the bush of what was once Zululand, difficult to find, easy to miss. More a squatters' camp than a village, it nevertheless offers a shabby air of permanence, with at least a hundred or so Zulus residing in corrugated tin shacks and cardboard shanties, all either on their way to someplace else or with no other place to go.

The land around it bristles with monuments marking its violent past, but in the village itself there is not the slightest whiff of history. No one can say when it was settled. No one seems to know who arrived first or if any of the original families remain. It simply sits there in undistinguished anonymity on a low rise beneath a few scraggly trees, several miles from the nearest highway, almost invisible from the sun-baked ruts of a nearby secondary road. It is so wretched a place that if one day it were to be utterly destroyed by some mighty force of nature— by flood or fire, by earthquake or storm—only the immediate survivors would know or care that it had ever been there at all; and eventually, after the passing of a few seasons, when the rains and the winds had swept the little hill, even those who had lived there would not easily find it again, would not quickly point to the precise spot where once they had given birth to their babies and buried their dead.

Years after leaving it, one former resident of the village would simply recall that "it was a long way to go to some other place."

Others had more specific memories of crisp, clear mornings when only the birds were up and about earlier than the residents, of rosy dawns and kaleidoscopic dusks, of nights brilliantly illuminated by stars, deeply silent save for the snoring of the elderly or the crying of the infants or the naughty giggling of the older children—and occasionally, from somewhere out in the darkness, the cackling shriek of hyenas or the hoarse cough of a lonely leopard.

Yet those who remember such minute details about the village where the boy would be born cannot recall whether they were ever happy when they were living there or whether, when they left, they were sad to be going. People were always arriving or departing from the village, moving in or moving on. For one reason or another, they would awaken one morning, pack up and, leaving nothing of themselves behind, plod up the next long hill toward the smoky horizon, their meager belongings on their backs, in search of some other inhospitable piece of African real estate that no one else would have, where no one else would live, where no one given a choice—including the boy—would choose to be born.

His grandmother, Ruth Khumalo, had come to the village as a young girl. It was in the fifties or early sixties, she would recall, though she could not remember exactly how old she had been when she arrived with her mother and the rest of her large family, though not her father, whom she did not know and had never met. After leaving the Bantustan, they had lived on a succession of illegal sites—squatters' camps—some of which they had been forced to abandon, some of which they had left of their own volition, either in desperation or in the false hope of finding something better. They were not alone, of course. The migration of millions of black South Africans, begun by the British a half century before, had been accelerated by the land seizures of the Afrikaner government.

In retrospect it seems odd and, of course, tragic that in those days, just after World War II, while much of the rest of the world was at least tentatively coming to grips with the embarrassing inequities of racism and colonialism, the Afrikaners were moving their country headlong in the opposite direction. As a system of government, apartheid was designed to establish as a legal, philosophical, and theological proposition that black people, like Ruth Khumalo and her family—the vast majority of the population—were inferior human beings, incapable of participating in a civilized society, forever destined to be dependent on whatever the tiny white minority might benevolently offer them.

For all her life, Ruth had known nothing but this world—the world of apartheid, with its miasmic atmosphere of helplessness and hopelessness. Any other environment would have been totally foreign to her, perhaps even frightening. She could neither read nor write, had never been to school, never been to a hospital or a clinic or a dentist, had never had a new dress or owned a pair of shoes, had gone to bed hungry on more nights than she could remember, and, like millions of other black South Africans, she had learned to settle for what was there and to expect nothing more.

That was another by-product of apartheid—the disallowance of dreams. Faced with a vast void that represented both their past and their future, Ruth and other young girls in the village and thousands of others around the country fashioned their own alternate version of happiness in one pregnancy after another.

Beginning while she was still a teenager, Ruth would bear a number of children. She was never formally married. By then, that was not at all unusual among rural Zulu women. In a way, many thousands of them were simply practicing polygamy in reverse, minus the traditional protection and assistance of husbands and without the sense of family that had once been the strength of the tribe.

Her daughter, Daphne, was born in 1969 when Ruth was nineteen years old, the second or third of her children—their birth order was never made clear to me by anyone in the family. Like Ruth's childhood, Daphne's would be difficult. She would know only deprivation. Unlike her mother, however, Daphne went to school. Though it was not much of a school, it was still a school, and she learned to read and to write and to count. In most other respects, her life was a replication of her mother's—endless seasons and cycles of hopelessness and, by the time she was sixteen, pregnancy. In 1985, Daphne gave birth to a baby girl she named Mbali.

D aphne's second baby occupied so little space in her womb
that strangers in the village might not have noticed she
was pregnant at all. Even by December of 1988, when she told
her mother, Ruth, and her sisters and friends that she thought
she was probably in her eighth month, they all laughed at
her, found it hard to believe she was that far along, teased her
mercilessly about her size—or, more precisely, about her lack
of size.

Her younger half sister, Cynthia, remembered such moments.

How you do that, girl?

How come you not a cow like the rest of us?

You sleep with a midget?

Or some kind of alien?

You got a pea in your pod?

Girl, how you do that?

Like her mother, Daphne was a small but solidly constructed woman with an almost perfectly round face. But
while Ruth seemed congenitally dour, Daphne had a quick
smile and a sunny disposition, and most of the time she simply
laughed off the steady stream of jibes about her pregnancy, accepted them as just a bit of fun being poked within the bounds
of friendship and family.

Yet, as Cynthia would later remember, there was a limit to
her Daphne's patience.

Girl, where you get this child?

That question, which seemed invariably to follow the

others, was different for Daphne. She resented it, and it always seemed to set her teeth on edge—though if she'd heard
it once, she'd heard it a hundred times, so often in fact that her
daughter, just learning to talk, had eagerly enlisted in the in-
terrogation.

"Mummy?" Mbali would ask, splaying her chubby fingers
against Daphne's abdomen. "Where you get baby?"

Daphne always answered softly, "Just like you, this baby
comes from God."

To the others she offered not a word, for she knew that the
question was unrelated to biology, to where babies come from
and how they're made. They were not sophisticated teenage
girls, not by Western standards, but there had been no mystery
about sex and procreation for them since soon after they
had entered puberty. Many of them knew exactly what intercourse entailed and understood its potential for both pleasure
and pregnancy. Some had experimented with the enjoyment,
while others, like Daphne, had experienced both—and in the
nameless village where they all lived, neither was taboo. In
fact, both in their small world and in the larger swath of rural
South Africa, there were few if any role models for chastity,
including Daphne's mother.

Ruth seemed rather proud of the sexual choices she had
made in her life, did not regret them at all or regard them
as any different from those her own mother or her peers
had made. She defended them as customary, and as evidence
she declared that offhand she could not remember any marriages at all between the members of her extended family.
Nor could she identify a genuine couple among any of her

acquaintances—that is, a man and woman living under the same roof, committed to one another, regardless of their legal status. I once asked if she could explain why marriage or the tradition of couples seemed so unimportant to her and in her community. She shrugged and, after a moment's thought, turned the question in on itself. "Because it is not important," she growled, increasingly irritated with my prying. "And it never has been," she added. That would be her final word on the subject.

For Ruth this was simply the way it was, and just as she had incurred no condemnation, neither would Daphne face any cultural or moral indictment for having had her first baby at sixteen—"out of wedlock," as the Western euphemism would describe it—or for being pregnant again three years later and still unmarried.

Girl, where you get this child?

So if the question was not about biology, neither was it about deviating from the norm. Daphne was conforming to the standards and customs of her time and place, of her family, of her mother. She might be teased, but she would not be criticized.

Girl, where you get this child?

It wasn't a question of morality or cultural values. Her sisters and friends simply wanted to know the father's name—and her stony silence on the subject, as Cynthia recalled, served only to sharpen their probing.

We know it's Mbali's father.

The same man.

It has to be.

It's someone else?

A local fellow?

A Madadeni boy?

Do we know him?

Or that skinny kid from Osizweni?

You liked him, didn't you?

You said you did.

Tell us girl, where you get this child?

Only once did Daphne drop the veil, and then only on her own terms.

No, she told Cynthia, the father of her new baby was not the father of Mbali.

"Do I know him?" Cynthia had pressed.

Maybe, Daphne had answered.

"Tell me," Cynthia insisted, sensing a breakthrough. "I won't tell anybody else."

Yes you will.

"No I won't. I promise."

You have to. You can't help it.

Cynthia was forced to admit then and later that her half sister probably had a point.

Daphne's classroom education may have ended after the eighth grade, but she clearly grasped the sociological dynamics of their village. Primarily, the village lay within the economic sphere of the small town of Dannhauser; then, slightly farther away there was Dundee, which was a bit larger, and, beyond that, the city of Newcastle—the smoky coal-mining center named by the British for its counterpart in England—

and the nearby black townships of Madadeni and Osizweni. Compared to them, Daphne's nameless little village was utterly bland and boring. In such a place, so compact and so insular, privacy was minimal and gossip compulsive— which was why she had told Cynthia she would be unable to resist passing along her secret, *if* she knew the secret.

"We all loved to tittle-tattle," Cynthia would later explain. "All of us except Daphne. For some reason—I don't know why —she hated it. Just hated it."

Yet she could not escape it.

That previous winter—summer in America and Europe— when Daphne had returned from a brief stay in Johannesburg, having left Mbali in Ruth's care, she confessed she was disappointed not to have found either a job or a more promising life. Like so many black South Africans before her, she had discovered that her reach exceeded her grasp. Still, she said, she had not regretted the experience, and what she appreciated most about the big city was the anonymity it offered. She had simply vanished into its masses, and because no one had known who she was, no one had cared who she was. Everyone had left her alone, and she had liked it a lot, she said.

She told Cynthia she sometimes felt invisible there.

"But weren't you lonely?" her half sister asked. "I mean, sometimes?"

Yes, sometimes.

"Ha!" Cynthia chortled. "It's somebody from Johannesburg."

Who someone?

"This baby's father."

Uncharacteristically, Daphne snapped at her sister.

Leave me alone!

Her attitude puzzled her peers. As Cynthia would explain, a certain candor about such matters was an integral part of their fellowship in a place where they had so little else to entertain them. Besides, as her friends often pointed out, hadn't Daphne willingly identified Mbali's father even before she was born—and afterward had she not given her new daughter his surname? So why was she constructing and maintaining such a deep mystery about her second pregnancy?

Even all these years later, it remains a question—one of those to which I found no answer. Was she, like any other adolescent craving attention, simply encouraging more questions by refusing to answer any? Or had she simply had enough of people poking around in what she considered to be her business and hers alone? Cynthia did not regard Daphne as promiscuous—not in the context of their culture, at least—but she did admit to having entertained the possibility that Daphne would not *say* who the father was because she might not *know* who the father was.

Or could it have been that in December 1988, even in such a permissive time and place, Daphne suspected that she had somehow managed to cross a forbidden line into a social or cultural or family territory that was taboo?

For whatever reason, she kept the name of her new baby's father to herself. She had told Cynthia that he was not the father of her daughter, and Cynthia had believed her, had thought that was probably logical, since she had not seen that fellow

around since long before Mbali's birth. The truth—whatever
the truth was—would forever remain Daphne's secret.

In the context of her experience, it would have made perfect
sense for Daphne to keep silent about her second baby's father because she knew from her experience not to expect his
presence or participation in her life or in the life of their child.
After all, she had completely lost contact with Mbali's father
long before her birth, did not know if he knew he had a daughter, did not anticipate that she would ever see him again, and
frankly did not care if she did or not.

The same was true for *her* own father. She might have seen
him every single day on the road between her village and Madadeni or Dannhauser, but she would have had no idea who he
was, not even if he had happened to stroll into their dilapidated
shack one day and introduce himself. Similarly, her Zulu grandfathers were invisibly anonymous—and because there had never
been any constant male presence in her life, certainly not one
with any lasting significance for her, it was almost as though her
entire family, including her mother, actually had *come from God,*
conceived without benefit of male parents.

Paternity had been reduced to a triviality in the Zulu culture. Like marriage, the currency of fatherhood had been seriously devalued. At any age it was entirely acceptable—and
indeed much more the rule than the exception—for a man to
have intercourse with a woman without having to concern
himself with whether conception might occur. If a pregnancy

did result, which was quite often the case, since very few Zulu men or women practiced any form of birth control (like most African men, Zulus seemed to abhor the use of condoms), he would move blithely on, without a backward glance.

The old Zulu traditions of strong marriages and healthy families had faded into obsolescence. Like the colorful costumes and crafts of the past, they had become quaint if charming relics, not concepts with which Daphne was at all familiar. And who could blame her for concluding, having had no contact at all with her own father or her grandfathers and having already lost track of Mbali's father, that the father of the child growing inside her was similarly irrelevant to her life? He simply did not matter, and if he did not matter, why bother with his name?

Like millions of other black South Africans, Daphne had learned not to dream, had learned, as her mother had learned, to be realistic, to settle quietly for the way things were, for the way they had always been before, and for the way she was certain they would always be in her life, in her little settlement, in what had once been Zululand, in a country that would forever be ruled and run by whites.

"Is he a Zulu?" Cynthia had once asked her—and for once Daphne had given her a straight answer.

Yes, he is a Zulu man.

That seemed slightly important to both girls. After all, one in five black South Africans was a Zulu, by far the largest ethnic group in the population. Yet the years had worn down what had once been an enormous tribal pride. The most feared and fearsome people in all of southern Africa were by then famous

for little more than fierce outbursts of primitive political violence and a certain tourist appeal, which included Shaka Land,
a former movie set converted into a theme park and named
for their most famous chief. One Zulu writer suggested that
many of the more visible members of the tribe had by then become "postcard Zulus," merely costumed actors playing roles
they neither appreciated nor understood.

By December 1988, what was left of their land had become a fertile garden of cyclical poverty. It was as though their
privation was somehow genetic, transferred biologically in
some sad double helix of DNA from one Zulu generation to
the next. For Daphne and her friends, there was not much else
to expect from their lives except broken and usually dysfunctional families and perhaps a passing romance or two with a
man who would afterward promptly go on his way.

On the fourth day of February, 1989, Daphne rather
calmly announced that her water had broken and her
labor had begun. There was no hectic hurrying and scurrying
here and there. Having babies, after all, was not exactly a
novel event in the Khumalo family or in the lives of the other
families around them. As the usual afternoon thunderstorms
began to roil up on the horizon, someone rushed to a nearby
shebeen, a beer hall down the rutted road, to use the telephone there to call a relative who lived in the area. He came
quickly in the old truck he used to deliver firewood and, in
the pouring rain, drove Daphne to a rudimentary clinic in
Dannhauser. It was exclusively for black people, of course. Its

facilities were meager, its staff limited (there were no doctors on duty), and its hygiene suspect, but it was the same place where Mbali had been delivered hale and hearty by a midwife three years before—and late that evening, with the same woman in attendance, Daphne gave birth to the boy.

Early the next morning, after barely any sleep, cradling him in her arms and wearing the same clothes she had worn to the clinic, Daphne climbed into her relative's rickety truck again and took the bone-jarring ride back to the muddy settlement where, in addition to the usual clucking over a newborn and the predictable comparisons of his looks with those of his mother and grandmother (not to his anonymous father, of course), there was also a sudden comprehension of why Daphne had gained so little weight throughout her pregnancy.

The baby was tiny.

He weighed, Cynthia would guess, no more than four or five pounds, if that, and he was clearly not nearly as healthy as his sister, Mbabli, had been as an infant. His nasal passages were clogged, his breathing severely labored.

"It'll take a lot of sucking for that boy," Ruth noted sadly as Daphne sat outside the shack, nursing him in the afternoon sun.

Mbali stood nearby, wide-eyed. She approached her mother and tentatively touched her brother's face. "Mummy?" she asked. "Where you get this baby?"

As always, Daphne answered softly, *Just like you, this baby comes from God.*

Mbali asked his name.

Daphne thought for a moment, then answered.

This baby's name is Xolani and, just like you, Nkosi. See? Mbali Nkosi. Xolani Nkosi. Just the same.

Everyone assumed, of course, that her secret was at last a secret no more. She had given the boy her daughter's surname. Therefore, his father and the girl's were one and the same. Case closed. Cynthia thought she knew better but was not quite certain. Daphne had told her that Mbali's father was *not* the father of the child she had been carrying.

"So why give him the same name?" Cynthia asked.

It's for Mbali. Now they can really be a brother and sister. Not half, like us.

The identity of his father would remain Daphne's secret, another of the questions to which I could not find an answer. Yet, whoever he was, Daphne was quite mistaken about his unimportance or his irrelevance to her life. In fact, whoever he may have been, or whatever she may have thought of him, or whatever the circumstances of their relationship, or however dear or trivial he may have been to her or she to him—in terms of her life and her survival, he was the most significant person she had ever met or known in her life—or ever would.

He had introduced into her young body something much more vital than his semen. He had impregnated her with death.

Daphne was not yet twenty years old, yet she was already dying—and on the very first day of his life, so was her son, the tiny child who had occupied so little space inside her womb.

TWO

In South Africa many years ago, I met a woman I will always remember. Though I never knew her name, I changed her life.

In the early 1980s, on one of my first trips to the country, along with a producer and a camera crew, I was working on a variety of stories, among them one that focused on whites actively opposed to the government's policies on race. One such courageous figure was Helen Suzman, the daughter of one of the country's most prominent families, a member of parliament, the founder of an antiapartheid group called the Black Sash, and a constant thorn in the government's side. Another renegade was Nadine Gordimer, the novelist whose brutally honest portraits of her country would eventually win her the Nobel Prize for Literature. In those days, however, they had brought her the condemnation of many fellow whites in her native land.

In preparation for our interview, I had purchased her latest novel from the gift shop of my hotel in downtown Johannesburg. It was the last copy on the shelf. I read it over the course of a couple of nights, then gave it to the producer and the cameraman and took it along for her autograph, and while we enjoyed a leisurely afternoon tea in her living room, she kindly inscribed it for me. Afterward, back at the hotel and still carrying Ms. Gordimer's novel, I stopped off in the gift shop to pick up the newspapers. The black woman behind the counter rang them up and, noticing the book under my arm, asked that I hand it over so that she could check its price as well. I told her I had purchased it earlier. Not possible, she said, because this particular book had only arrived that morning. I looked at the shelf and, sure enough, there were several new copies of the novel in stock. But when I tried to explain to her what I thought had happened—that the shop had sold out and the local distributor had sent along a few more copies—she was adamant.

I decided not to argue any further. Instead I gave her only the price of the newspapers, walked out of the shop with the book still under my arm, and took the elevator up to my room. It was a mistake that would have dire consequences. A few minutes later, there was a knock on my door. The manager of the hotel—a white man, of course—was waiting in the hallway and, just behind him, the black woman from the gift shop. She seemed quite nervous. I was surprised that the manager had known where to find me but, in those days, I was still rather naïve about South African attitudes toward the foreign press.

"This girl here says," he began, nodding back over his shoulder toward the woman who was clearly not a girl, "you forgot to pay for a book you took. I'm sure it's a mix-up, and I wanted to see if we could straighten it out."

I invited him in and, while the woman remained in the hall, repeated the explanation I'd offered her downstairs. I showed him not only Ms. Gordimer's dated inscription but also the purchase receipt from several days before, retained so that I could submit the cost of it to my network as part of my expenses. It was an airtight alibi. I was exonerated. The manager backed his way out of the room, offering a litany of apologies. Even through the closed door, I could hear his angry voice as he hustled the young woman back to the elevators. A benign incident had taken an ugly turn.

In a few minutes, a bellman arrived at my door with champagne, a box of chocolates, and a cordial note from the manager, reiterating his apologies. I immediately called down but was told he had left for the evening and would be unavailable until the following day. The next morning, when I stopped by the gift shop for the newspapers, the woman was not behind the counter. I went straight to the hotel's executive offices, where the manager told me she was no longer on his staff.

Wholly unjustified, I said. "She made an honest mistake, and nobody's the worse for it," I added.

With considerable venom in his voice, the manager said,

"That girl will never work here again, and she will never work in any hotel in Johannesburg."

I asked her name.

"Unimportant," he said.

I demanded her name.

"Offhand, I don't know it."

I was incredulous—and angry. "You just fired her. How could you not know her name?"

"Because it doesn't matter—and this, sir, is not your business. The matter is finished."

Short of fisticuffs he seemed to be right. It was finished.

South Africa was that sort of place and had been for a long time—a country where, for generation after generation, millions upon millions of black men and women and children were penalized and persecuted simply for their genes, for their biological heritage, for their involuntary membership in one particular component of the human race—and as a routine part of their penalty, they were robbed of their individual identities. That the hotel manager claimed not to know the woman's name should not have come as a surprise to me or anyone else. For many of the whites in charge of the country, either the government or some hotel, black people were quite literally nameless—and, in a sense, from Cairo to Cape Town, that has been the fate of most black Africans wherever they happen to live. If it has not always been the purposeful product of racism or bigotry, it does not much matter. What does matter is that in much of the rest of the world—the white world in particular—all these millions of human beings lack any specific identity, and as a result they are accorded no dignity or respect. They are quite simply all the same, a dark mass of people whose names are not important.

My own limp means of compensating —much like a bottle of champagne and a box of chocolates—is to have become something of a name freak, especially when I'm in Africa, but also just about anywhere else I travel in the developing world. Whomever I meet, I always insist on his or her name, and if it's difficult to say—as it quite often is—I always demand a lesson in pronunciation. It means next to nothing, of course, but it is my way of reminding myself that there was once an African woman whose life I inadvertently changed yet who was for me as nameless as Daphne's village, as anonymous as the father of the baby who had occupied so little space in her womb.

In those days the country was understandably awash with secrets. After all, it is quite impossible for a police state run by a tiny minority to impose its will on a vast majority without hiding much of what it does. Nor can those who oppose such a government—who seek its overthrow by one means or another, including by acts of violence often described as terrorism—succeed or survive without deception and camouflage. Yet in those first few months of Xolani's life in his mother's arms and in her village, no secret was more critical to South Africa's future than were a series of covert negotiations between representatives of the apartheid government and the man who had been for so long the personification of its enemies.

Imprisoned for nearly thirty of his seventy years—including twenty on Robben Island, the Alcatraz of South Africa Nelson Mandela had been all but invisible for longer than Daphne had been alive (the last new photograph of him had been published in 1965), had been a prisoner since Ruth was barely a teenager. Still, with the possible exception of Muhammad Ali, he was the most famous black man on earth. As Anthony Sampson, his biographer, would write, he had survived long enough to become "the last great freedom fighter." International icon or not, however, in early 1989, while Daphne and Mbali and Xolani and the rest of her family remained captives of apartheid, Mandela remained a prisoner of the South African government—though his status had changed dramatically in the previous few weeks. In December he had been transferred from a hospital where he had been treated for tuberculosis to a prison complex near Cape Town, installed in a comfortable bungalow with a garden and pool, and provided with a friendly white warder who cooked his meals and cleaned his rooms.

Moreover, he had been driven to several face-to-face meetings with a small cadre of government officials desperate to resolve the conditions apartheid had created in their country. The Afrikaners knew they had shot themselves in the foot. After more than a decade of increasingly violent protests and turbulence in the townships—ignited by student uprisings in Soweto, then fueled by the Black Consciousness Movement led by Steven Biko—matched by increasingly murderous repression from the government, the tension in the country was nearly palpable. If the black liberationists had not overthrown the white government, neither had the government squashed their resistance or persuaded them or the rest of the world of the legitimacy of its power. Allistair Sparks, one of the country's most distinguished journalists, described the country as having reached "a state of violent equilibrium."

The Afrikaners had tried to pacify the hordes of black people they governed but did not rule, had pumped millions of dollars into the townships, had co-opted Zulus and other black leaders with promises of prosperity and status; still the jails were flooded with protesters, and the violence continued. In 1988, the year before the boy was born, there had been 115 executions. Only three of those put to death had been white. South African agents had assassinated black activists in Mozambique, in Botswana, even as far away as Paris. Nothing had worked, and many of the most recalcitrant racists in positions of power were admitting, only to themselves if not to each other, that without substantial change the country would explode in an all-out civil war or, with the sanctions imposed on it, would implode economically—or perhaps both, simultaneously.

Mandela was an old man, but he was clearly their best and quite probably their last chance. So in those first few months of the boy's life, in a variety of secret locations, the talks had begun and continued, with the future of South Africa hanging on their success or their failure. Mandela knew that the apartheid government had blinked, had decided to resolve the unbearable tensions in the country by doing what its leaders had sworn never to do—to negotiate with him. Few South Africans beyond the small circle of those involved in the talks knew what was going on, certainly not Daphne and Ruth and Cynthia, who went about their hard lives in a village that seemed to have no secrets at all, since everyone was by then convinced that they knew the identity of Xolani's father.

That Nkosi fellow, they all agreed—but they never saw him around. Indeed, they seldom saw any men around the village.

On one of my first assignments in South Africa, I was struck by the scarcity of young and middle-aged men in many of the villages I visited. Most of the visible males were children, young teenagers, and elderly men. Even to someone as new to the country and as green as I was then, it was obvious. When I asked where all the men were, the women always said they were working.

Where?

Away.

That was the truth. Ever since the British had forced those millions of black men into their mines and mills, to be exploited as an inexpensive labor force in the dangerous and backbreaking business of extracting the country's subterranean treasures, the men had been steadily vanishing from the countryside. Some may have found jobs as gardeners or handymen, houseboys or drivers or farmhands working on acreage that had once belonged to them or their ancestors; and some of the black women may have tried to make ends meet as poorly paid domestics in white households, as maids or nannies or cooks; but for most of the rest of them, it was the mines and the mills. If the men did not happen to reside near them, they had gone to where the jobs were.

Over several generations this had evolved into one of South Africa's most telling and tragic statistical patterns: vast numbers of black men leaving their rural homes and their families for employment in some faraway place. The mining companies built crude hostels for them, squalid single-sex dormitories, while the government, understandably anxious about such large concentrations of black men, had enacted those Draconian pass laws, a series of residency requirements that complicated or generally eliminated most freedom of movement. Once having relocated at a particular mine or mill in a particular locale, it was difficult for black men to travel back and forth, to and from their original homes, except for occasional visits. Eventually an entirely new social structure was built and rigidly enforced. Miles from their roots, many of the men created separate lives for themselves. Some sent back small portions of their meager earnings, but many went on about their business, cut off from their previous lives and re-sponsibilities, whatever the strength of their emotional ties. Many began to anesthetize themselves with bad sorghum beer, and many visited the diseased prostitutes tolerated or in some cases provided by the companies. Thousands of men moved in with thousands of local women, siring thousands of children whose needs consumed whatever money their displaced fa-thers were earning or were perhaps willing to pay, leaving little or nothing at all for the women and children the men had left behind.

It was a cultural catastrophe—and yet, for the women in the village where Ruth and Daphne and Cynthia and the boy lived, it was simply a fact of life, like the thunderstorms that invariably boiled up on summer afternoons. There was nothing they could do about either the weather or the absence of responsible men. In a way Nelson Mandela was one of them. He was not around and had not been for years—and whether he was then in prison or in a hospital or in a comfortable house with a white man preparing his meals did not much matter to them. What did or did not happen to him was of little consequence in their lives or in the lives of the others who lived alongside them in the dirt-poor desperation of the village. Their closest connection to him was mere coincidence. All those years before, Mandela had been arrested and taken into custody in a town not far from where they all lived, although they did not know even that small fact of South African history. In fact, Mandela was rarely mentioned by any of them.

It wasn't that they were totally unaware or unconcerned with what had been happening in their country; it was simply that they were rural people who lived their lives separate and apart from the trauma and turmoil of the troubled townships. Except for occasional excursions into them—in Daphne's case to the school in Madadeni—they were not much involved, certainly not actively enlisted in the ongoing insurrection that had captured the outside world's interest and imagination. Among her family and her friends, the focus was on surviving from one day to the next—and there did not seem to be any possible escape from that rhythm and routine, which had been precisely the white government's objective with its imposition of apartheid some forty years before.

Not that Zulus were the only targets. For all those years, the system had hammered every nonwhite in the country: Tswanas, Xhosas (Mandela's tribe), Vendas, Tsongas, and an assortment of other ethnic communities, along with Asians and coloreds (those of mixed racial parentage) as well. A couple of generations of such official madness had effectively separated most nonwhites from any hope of progress or self-improvement, whether through education or connections or circumstances or pure luck. Slavery and the slave trade had long been banished, of course, yet black South Africans like Daphne's family were subject to a system and practice of twentieth-century bondage no less cruel, no less repressive, with no realistic promise of relief and no prospect of emancipation.

They could not own property of any significant value, and regardless of the legitimacy of the title or deed they presented, they were legally unable to hold on to any land claimed by whites. They could not live in areas other than those specifically designated for them by the government, mainly in the townships or in the Bantustans or in fetid squatters' camps or primitive rural settlements. Whatever their instincts or however deep their anger with the status quo, they could not legally belong to any organization or political party that espoused, endorsed, or otherwise encouraged the concept of racial equality. They could not move freely about their own country. They could not vote. In effect they were not citizens at all. They were strictly forbidden to do anything—in public, at least—that did not have the prior approval of a white regime ferociously devoted to their continued servitude. For the slightest deviation, the smallest violation, they could, like Nelson Mandela, end up in prison—or worse.

Not that the system had stood unopposed, unchallenged over the years, but all the mass demonstrations, strikes, sickouts, even episodes of armed rebellion had had little impact on the government or on the hearts and minds of those committed to its racist canons. The greater the resistance, the greater the retaliatory force against it. As it had when the British had stifled the Zulus' tax rebellion, the government still had most of the weapons. There had been several generations of vigorous opposition to apartheid. There had been thousands of casualties. Nothing much had changed.

Daphne and Cynthia and their mother, Ruth, and all their friends were the offspring of this static era, the children of a system so mean, so ugly but so deeply entrenched that only a few South Africans, black or white or colored, could imagine anything else. It was no wonder that so many of the young Zulu girls focused more on boys and babies than on dreams of a different life.

Perhaps, if someone had asked her or urged her, Daphne might have given herself to something other than a man who would quickly vanish from her life. She might have become part of the protests and demonstrations, might have found meaning for her existence in the liberation struggle. But Zulu political leaders were not fond of Mandela or his organization—the African National Congress—and many had, in fact, divorced themselves from him and its efforts. Instead they were energetically and often violently promoting the Inkatha Freedom Party, mainly Zulu in membership, making their own deals with the government, in pursuit of their own separate peace.

So Daphne had not manned the barricades, had not marched on the police stations, had not hurled rocks or insults at constables with shotguns. She had never seen, much less raised her voice or a challenging fist at, a "hippo," the armored personnel carrier used by the South African military and police. She had never tasted tear gas or fled in panic from a barrage of gunfire aimed at ending this protest or that demonstration. No one she knew had ever been wounded, much less killed, and among her acquaintances none had disappeared into the dreaded invisibility of the jails or the prisons. Although racial unrest had by then become an unpleasant reality in South Africa, it all remained rather dim and distant for Daphne.

The much more important concern for her, for her family, and for her neighbors was the hand-to-mouth survival they had endured all their lives. They cared little for the right to vote or to own property or for a good education available to all. What really mattered was tending to the tiny, scraggly gardens in which they grew a bit of their food, gathering bundles and bales of firewood for sale or for the next day's cooking, hiking several miles to a well or a spigot and then hauling the foul water back in heavy jerry cans balanced on their heads. Their meals were prepared over outdoor fires, and after sparse dinners they slept on mattresses made of straw or simply pallets made of filthy blankets. They had neither electricity nor plumbing. They were without toilets or television sets or telephones. They washed their faded clothing in steaming black kettles and draped it on rocks to be dried by the sun. They owned no cars, no trucks, no tractors. They had no easy access to doctors and none at all to dentists. They often paid *inyanga*s or *songoma*s—traditional healers—for treatment or advice about their health.

Public education was a cruel joke. The schools were unworthy of the name, and, like Daphne and later Cynthia, most young people who did attend, at some point in their teens or sometimes even earlier, simply walked away, barely literate if that, from the crude, crowded classrooms.

As far as they knew, nobody cared.

Nelson Mandela might be a hero, a man to respect and to follow. He might be famous the world over. He might be conducting secret negotiations with the government, might be released from prison someday, might lead black South Africans into their freedom in a new country, but for Daphne and her family and her friends, none of that mattered much.

In that February of 1989, what mattered to her was the future of her little girl, and more important, her newborn son—and for Daphne his future was measured by hours and days, not weeks and months.

As the months of 1989 passed, Daphne realized with a deadening sadness that the boy was ill—very ill—and not getting better. His breathing had not noticeably improved. His nasal passages were still seriously clogged. His adenoids and tonsils were swollen, and the inside of his mouth was blistered. He had a chronic cough, was constantly snorting and snuffling, ate and nursed sparingly, but what alarmed Daphne most was that he had gained almost no weight. Indeed, it sometimes seemed to her that he was shrinking right before her eyes.

Her instincts toward him were tender and generous, but something had already happened to her little boy, something that merely a name, however lovingly given, could not reverse, something a good mother's attention and concern could neither help nor change. It had already happened to thousands of babies all across southern Africa and continues to happen to them even now. Although I did not see the boy when he was still an infant in Daphne's arms, I'm reasonably confident I know exactly what he must have looked like, having seen so many like him.

One of them occupies a particularly vivid place in my memory.

On a steamy morning in Gaborone, the capital of Botswana—a small country just next door to South Africa—as I accompanied a young pediatrician on his rounds through the children's ward of Princess Marina Hospital, the city's main health facility, I came face to face with Kebo, a sad-looking little guy, wailing ferociously in his crib, peering through its bars with eyes as big as saucers, in search of his mother.

From his size I judged his age to be about a year.

"No," said the doctor. He picked up a chart at the end of the crib and pointed. "Look, he's past two."

I said I didn't see how he could be, given how terribly small he was.

"The wasting, the stunting, is typical," he said. "He won't get much bigger than this before . . . before he dies."

I asked when that might be.

The young doctor shrugged. "Not long," he said.

I had also seen Kebo's mother earlier that day, or rather seen her lifeless form wrapped in a blanket on a gurney being rolled through one of the hospital corridors, headed toward the morgue in the rear of the building. Thandie Kabelo was twenty-six—and although her name was spoken often the next day when she was buried in the hard, dark earth near Artesia, the village where she had been born, the name of the disease that had killed her was never once mentioned, not by her friends or the members of her extended family who had gathered for her funeral, not by her mother, and not by her other two children—her ten-year-old daughter and six-year-old son—who had survived her. Although seven other residents of the village had died that year and another three or four dozen were seriously ill, no one there knew what had killed Thandie or what was killing the rest of them.

Francinah Diehobe, a family-education worker in the village, explained that the mourners did not know the cause of Thandie's death "because we do not tell them." Doing the best she could with English, she said, "No, they do not know. We don't allow to tell the people what kind of disease the people died."

In those days—and even now to an alarming extent—medical professionals like Ms. Diehobe did not tell them because they understood from experience that the disease that had killed Thandie often transformed its victims and their families into social outcasts. Accordingly, it was more often than not referred to by any number of euphemisms— as simply "this" disease or "that" disease or "the thin disease" or "the whore's disease" or, because they may have heard it mentioned in broadcasts, "the radio disease." In some locales, though no one could say just why, it was called "the grid disease" or "Z3."

It was rarely called what it was: AIDS.

Consequently, Thandie never knew the name of the disease that had made her so ill, that had tainted and fouled her blood and ravaged and reduced her body until it could no longer combat the slightest bacterial invasion from any source (at the hospital her death certificate listed "respiratory infection" as the cause)—and, perhaps mercifully, she would never know that she had unintentionally done what she would never have purposefully or consciously done. She had passed along the virus that would kill her to Kebo, her son, the little boy behind the bars of his crib, crying for a mother he would never see again, no matter how long he might survive.

By any name the disease had taken a new tack, one that epidemiologists in the West had not foreseen. In 1989, in Europe and in America, AIDS was still regarded mainly as a threat to homosexual men or, in some instances, drug addicts who shared their needles. There were, here and there, a few cases of infections caused by tainted transfusions of blood—Arthur Ashe, the international tennis star, would be one notable example; a child in Florida who was placed in a glass isolation booth in her classroom would be another—but health officials in most of the Western countries and especially in the United States saw these cases as anomalies and were primarily focused on gay male adults as the group most vulnerable to AIDS.

The statistics they saw seemed to buttress that judgment.

When Masters and Johnson, whose study and books on sexual practices in America had brought them considerable fame, published a report suggesting otherwise—asserting that heterosexuals were also vulnerable—they were more or less shouted down. For instance, Robert Gould, a prominent gynecologist in New York City, responded that the risk of AIDS to heterosexuals was so remote that healthy women need not take any precautions at all, a view given substantial and respectful coverage by the media. Even the highly publicized death from AIDS in December 1988 of Max Robinson, my notoriously straight colleague at ABC News, had seemed to change very few minds,

In Africa, however, history was in the process of changing all that.

Consider this: In the late 1980s, in a desolate stretch of famine-stricken Somalia (the descriptive words are probably redundant, since most of Somalia is desolate, and it has rarely not been famine-stricken), as I was being driven with a camera crew to a feeding station for refugees far out in the bush, I spotted what looked like an airstrip hidden behind a long, tall berm. We stopped and found row after row of old Soviet MiGs, perhaps as many as a hundred, all rusting and cannibalized, missing engines here and wings there, cockpits gone, stripped of armaments. They were rather pitiful monuments to the Cold War, which had been hotly contested in Africa by surrogates of the United States and the USSR—and fighter jets were not the only weapons generously supplied to the principal combatants. Over the previous couple of decades, millions of land mines and hand grenades and a variety of small arms had also been made available from Moscow and Washington to various African countries, either to prop up their governments or to destabilize them, depending on who was giving and who was getting. The assault rifle, usually the AK-47, had become as common a currency in some countries as camels or cattle. In many of those places, most of which had become independent in the previous twenty years, the presidents and government ministers who had first acquired power had been corrupted by the millions of dollars or rubles pouring into their coffers and had been reluctant to surrender their offices—and the enormous opportunities to line their own pockets—through democratic elections, no matter how unpopular their regimes. In many cases their governments were utter failures and poverty in these states was increasing astronomically. As a consequence of such deprivation and hardship combined with a long season of civil wars and revolutions, millions of refugees were created, and millions of them were trudging back and forth across borders and boundaries, looking for safe haven and survival—and companionship either permanent or fleeting.

AIDS was moving right along with them.

By 1989, the year Daphne's son was born, the scholars and scientists attending the 4th International AIDS Conference in Stockholm were estimating that about 5 million people in 130 countries were then carrying the virus, with about 150,000 suffering from the full-blown effects of the disease. That same year, in its final report of the decade, the World Health Organization predicted that by the end of the century, 5 million people would be suffering from the disease and 15 to 20 million would be infected. They had no idea how wrong they were. However well-meaning and deeply committed to finding a way to stop the scourge, they could not see then, could not even imagine then, what was happening in Africa. It was too far beneath their radar. Infections in Africa were already soaring at such a terrifying rate that Western estimates were miles behind the reality. Furthermore, in Africa AIDS had already become a disease not mainly of gay men or drug addicts but mainly of heterosexuals; moreover, it was rapidly becoming a woman's disease. And as it became a woman's disease, it became a children's disease as well. Inside their wombs or in their birth canals or through their milk, infected African women by the tens of thousands, including Thandie and Daphne, were unintentionally transmitting the AIDS virus to tens of thousands of their African babies, including Kebo—and Xolani Nkosi.

Daphne, however, did not know what was wrong with her son. She knew only that all through 1989, in the first months of his life, his physical condition continued to deteriorate. And although it would be a dramatic year for South Africa, she was not interested in much besides Xolani.

In July, Mandela met with President P. W. Botha, the hardline Afrikaner who was himself called "The Crocodile" and who had once called Mandela a terrorist and communist and vowed never to speak a single word to him. In August, after suffering a stroke, Botha resigned and was succeeded by F. W. de Klerk, who was formally elected to office in September. In October he ordered the release from prison of several notable allies of Mandela's. In December, Mandela and de Klerk sat down together—and there was much talk and considerable hope Mandela would soon be released.

But Daphne's detachment from such events was nearly complete. She knew next to nothing about any of them and cared less about what she did know. What she knew for certain was that her son was in jeopardy.

"He just never seemed to get any better," Cynthia remembered. "And also he wasn't growing much. He never really took much milk from Daphne. I don't know, he was just such a tiny little thing, and he was so sick all the time." There were few in the family, she said, or among the neighbors in the village, who had any confidence that the boy would survive 1989, much less live to see his first birthday that next February.

But somehow he did—perhaps it was the strength of his Zulu genes—and although his birthday was not a moment of great celebration in the village, it would almost perfectly coincide with the most unrestrained joy ever expressed in the streets of South Africa. Just two days before, on February 2, in a speech to Parliament, President de Klerk had repudiated apartheid, dismantled many of its restrictions, officially legalized the previously outlawed African National Congress, along with other protest groups, and ordered the release of all nonviolent political prisoners. Finally he promised that Mandela himself would soon be unconditionally released—and he kept his word.

Exactly one week after Xolani's first birthday, the old man walked out of jail. He was past seventy-one years old. More than half his life had been stolen from him by a succession of apartheid governments, but he was at last free. For the first time in two generations, South African newspapers published his photograph, splashed it all over their front pages, as did nearly every other paper in the world, and television broadcasts around the globe were filled with the images of his release and the wild celebrations that followed.

For several years the country had been teetering dangerously at the edge of an abyss. Neither Mandela nor anyone else knew whether the strength of his character or the myth and magic of his presence would be sufficient to bring South Africa back from the brink, to give it an opportunity to survive and prosper as a civilized nation, to give all its children—including Xolani Nkosi— a chance to fill their lungs with the breath of freedom instead of the noxious stench of apartheid.

But the jubilation that spread through the townships and across much of the country failed to reach the remote settlement where Daphne and her son lived.

"Of course we knew who Mandela was," Cynthia said, "and we were glad he was no longer in jail, but we weren't sitting around thinking the world was now going to be a better place or that our lives would be a lot better now that he was free."

And Daphne, she recalled, "cared only about the baby, that's all. Nothing else mattered to her. It was all she ever talked about. She had to find a way to make him better." And, said Cynthia, she seemed quite sad. "She just hardly laughed at all, not like she used to."

Daphne had tried everything, and nothing had worked. Finally, given the absence of any promising medical treatment and assistance in the place where she and the boy lived, she decided they would have to live in some other place. She would move, and by moving she would somehow find something better for herself and her children. She could measure the boy's decline, if not hour by hour, then at least day by day—the coughing, the congestion, the sore throat, the earaches, and the raspy rale in his sunken chest. She thought that if only she could find a reasonably decent location for them to live within reach of some modern medical facilities, perhaps there would be some hope for him.

Moreover, although she did not mention it to her mother, she did tell Cynthia she was a bit anxious about her own health. She seemed not to have the energy or the stamina she once had, seemed to grow extraordinarily tired in the middle of the day, long before what had to be done was done. "But," Cynthia remembered, "she said she was sure everything would be fine if she could just find somebody to help the baby."

Daphne had no idea what was happening to him or to her, but it is quite clear that she was absolutely determined to do what she believed had to be done for the sake of her baby. After all the dehumanization of apartheid, after the generations in which marriage and family and education and health and hope had been so badly eroded—after all that, the maternal instincts and devotion of one twenty-year-old Zulu woman were still strong.

Like the Kumalos' fictional son in Alan Paton's novel, the real-life Khumalo daughter would strike out for Johannesburg—in Zulu it was called Egoli, "the city of gold"—to find help for her son.

The simple plan she devised would probably have been familiar to thousands of young South African women of the time, for thousands of them were in similar if not identical circumstances and making similar plans to escape them. She would leave Mbali and Xolani in the care of their grandmother, Ruth, and the rest of her family in the settlement. She would catch a ride on a jitney bus, find a job of some sort and a place to live. Then, after she was settled in, she would return for the children and take them with her. "And she said that anybody else who wanted to could come with her, too," Cynthia recalled, "and I told her I probably would—and our mother said she didn't know, but maybe she would go, too."

Daphne departed late that winter—late summer in the Northern Hemisphere—in August or September, Cynthia said, carrying her meager belongings in a small cardboard suitcase, determined that this time Johannesburg would be different for her.

It was.

In a few weeks, she was hired as a sweeper and cleaner by a beauty salon in Benoni, a community on the eastern fringes of the city, not far from its sprawling international airport. She found two rooms in barely livable condition in a dilapidated

house on the road from Benoni to the township of Daveyton.
Despite her dwindling energy, she worked hard, carefully
saved her earnings, got by on one meal each day, scrupulously
paid her rent, and, in November or December, returned
to the settlement to find that her mother and Cynthia had
given some thought to her offer and had decided to come with
her back to Johannesburg, along with the children, Mbali and
the boy. The others in the family, if they chose, could follow later, Daphne told them. For the time being, there was
simply not enough space for everyone in the rooms she had
found. They would be cramped as it was. They said good-bye
to their friends and their kin, turned their backs on the mud
and dirt and grit and grime of the settlement, and were off,
the five of them. For generations it had been an altogether too
familiar sight in South Africa: another group of black migrants
on the road again, their earthly possessions on their backs,
searching once more for slightly better times in a slightly better place.

And for a brief while, it was better—until Daphne finally
managed to schedule appointments for herself and her son at
one of the city's hospitals.

I was not present, of course, and have no way of knowing
what took place when Daphne finally discovered why she
had been feeling so lethargic, why she always seemed to run
out of gas so soon every day—but I do know what it meant
to someone else at the moment the same explanation was
provided.

One morning, in a hospital in Malawi, in a tiny examination room just off a large ward overflowing with patients, most of them with AIDS—hundreds of dying men and women lay on blankets in every available space, in the aisles, under occupied beds butted up against each other—I stood in a corner and listened and watched as a physician sat down with a young black man to tell him his diagnosis. The patient looked to be in his mid-twenties, though it was difficult to tell exactly, since his entire appearance was haggard and his face was thin and drawn.

Outside on the lawn were hundreds of Malawians who had traveled miles from their outlying villages in the bush to stay with their relatives or to visit them for a while. They had set up camp on the hospital grounds. Smoke rose in wisps from small cooking fires, and the women stirred gruel in dirty pots and pans. Some of the men and boys were collecting firewood. Their laundry, washed in a nearby creek, hung on the branches of trees. Little gangs of noisy, naked children played in what had once been flower beds. Here and there, skinny dogs slunk from one family group to the next, begging breakfast.

Inside the examination room, the doctor—a white man from the Netherlands, come to work in Malawi as a volunteer—was perched on a wheeled stool, a clipboard in one of his hands. He rolled himself to within touching distance of the young man, laid his free hand on the man's knee, and delivered his verdict in roughly accented English. An interpreter standing nearby translated his words to the patient. I was leaning into a corner of the room, trying to make myself inconspicuous if not invisible, but watching and listening.

"You are very sick," the doctor began.

The young man nodded gravely, his eyes wide with apprehension.

"You have a very bad condition."

The young man said nothing.

"It is a condition of the blood."

The young man was silent but nodded again, just a slight movement of the head, almost imperceptible.

"Your condition is called AIDS," the doctor continued. "Do you know of this disease?"

The young man said yes, he was familiar with that name. "It is also the thin disease," he said.

"Yes," the doctor said. "Do you know what it means to have it? To have the thin disease?"

The young man said he did not really know but had heard and believed that it was very bad.

"Yes, that is correct. It is very bad, and it also means that there is nothing I can do for you."

The young man stared at the doctor.

"It means, I'm afraid, that you will not live much longer," the doctor said as gently as possible. "It means that you will not live to be an old man."

The young man took a deep breath and said he thought perhaps he had only a bad chest cold.

"Yes," said the doctor, "you do have a serious infection in your chest, but that is because of AIDS, because of the thin disease. Do you understand?"

The young man said he did understand, and suddenly his

face changed dramatically. What had been a blank mask, absent of emotion, became a portrait of fear. At last he spoke.

"So I am soon dying, yes?" he said.

The little room was silent, thick with the young man's bewildered sadness. Outside, the children seemed even noisier. A dog yelped, and just beyond the window, an ancient grandmother screamed at a wizened old fellow to remove a pot from their fire. The doctor rolled his stool closer, placed his clipboard on the floor, and put both his hands on the young man's knees.

"Yes, my friend," he said, "you are soon dying."

By that morning in 1999, more than a million people in Malawi—a tiny nation with a population of only 11 million— were infected with the virus, yet only thirty of them were receiving the triple-drug therapy of antiretroviral medications—the so-called cocktail—that had extended and enhanced thousands of lives in America and in Europe. Although the highest incidence of infection was among the country's more affluent and educated, the drugs, at an annual cost of about $10,000, were far beyond the incomes of the vast majority of them and certainly far beyond the reach of the young man in the little examination room. As many as half a million Malawians had already died of AIDS, and at least 7,000 had died in the first few months of 1999—and in the fifteen years since the first case had been diagnosed there, the disease had created nearly half a million orphans. Moreover, during that same period, the life expectancy for babies born in Malawi had been reduced to only thirty-six years.

The young man, of course, was unaware of these grim numbers, but he had heard from others that some people who were infected had actually been healed with a miracle recipe. In fact, thousands of infected Malawians were clamoring to scores of quick-money quacks for the magic cure.

"There is some kind of potion, isn't there?" he asked.

The doctor shook his head. "I'm afraid there is nothing, my friend," he said.

The young man clearly understood what he had heard from the doctor—and he had apparently heard enough. He slowly raised himself from his chair and, for some inexplicable reason, began feverishly brushing the front of his ragged clothing with the palms of his hands, as though in that way he might somehow rid himself of the diagnosis, the death sentence that had just been imposed on him. Finally he looked down at the doctor, still seated on his stool, and asked his permission to leave.

"Yes, of course," the doctor said, "but you are welcome to stay. There is not much room in the hospital, but we will try to find you a bed or one you can share or at least some blankets and a place on the floor. We have no medicine to give you, but I promise we will feed you each day and try to make you as comfortable as possible and try to keep your pain at a minimum."

The young man thanked him but declined the offer. He walked to the door, placed his hand on the knob, then stopped and turned back to the doctor.

"I will go home now," he said. "I will soon be dying at home."

Then he was gone.

The doctor in Johannesburg gave Daphne precisely the same diagnosis. He had examined her the week before and had taken blood from her for testing. She had returned for the results. He told her she had *ingculaza,* the Zulu word for AIDS. She knew what it meant and much later told Cynthia that she had not been all that surprised or shocked when the doctor had used that word. Neither of them was totally unaware of the disease. They had both heard it talked about in vague terms by some of the other young people they had met in Madadeni. Daphne knew that it had already killed some people there, and she had come to suspect that it was probably what was wrong with her, because the doctor who had examined the boy had already told her there was at least a possibility that his many illnesses were the result of an HIV infection—and if that turned out to be the case, though it was too soon to know for certain, then Daphne herself was quite probably infected. In fact, she told Cynthia after that appointment, "He said I might have given the sickness to Xolani."

For the moment, however, she told no one of the diagnosis. She'd heard what had happened to others whose infection had become public knowledge. Some had been attacked, several had been stoned, others had been forced from their houses and homes. The first woman in Cape Town to declare openly that she was infected had been found beheaded. Daphne was concerned enough about such potential threats to keep her diagnosis a secret.

It did not remain one for long. Sometime in the next month or so, the doctor who had told her of her condition called the

beauty salon where she worked and informed Daphne's employer of her condition. Almost immediately she was dis-
missed from her job. In another week or so, as word spread
through the neighborhood where she and her children and
Ruth and Cynthia were living, the five of them were summarily evicted from the two miserable rooms Daphne had rented.

"We begged the lady," Cynthia said, "but she wouldn't
change her mind. She said Daphne was too sick to live there,
and she thought probably the boy was, too, so we had to leave.
My mother was angry at the woman and spoke hard words to
her and called her many names, but Daphne just pleaded with
her and offered to clean her house for free if she would let us
stay. She still said no. I think she was afraid she would catch the
disease from Daphne or something. I think that's what everybody was afraid of. They didn't want to be anywhere near us."

For the next few days, sometimes with Cynthia at her side,
but more often alone, Daphne searched frantically for someplace else to live. She told her sister she felt it was her responsibility, since she had brought them all to Johannesburg. Finally
she found a vacant shack in a squatters' camp just outside
Daveyton, a township on the opposite side of the city from
Soweto. Once again they packed up the little they owned,
jammed themselves into a crowded jitney bus, and headed for
a place that would strike them as quite familiar—a collection
of matchbox shanties and mud daubed lean-tos with corrugated tin roofs held down by heavy stones. They moved into
one of them.

By then they were no longer looking for better times in a
better place. Johannesburg might have been the city of gold

for some, but for them—for Ruth and Cynthia and Daphne and Mbali and the boy—it had quickly become just another hopeless stop in the desperate journey of their lives, as bleak as the squalid settlement they had left behind them out in the bush of what had once been Zululand.

THREE

At the end of 1988, a three-hour drive from the wretched little village where Daphne was waiting for the birth of her son, another South African woman was living an entirely different life in an entirely different South Africa.

On a tree-lined street in one of Johannesburg's nicer neighborhoods, she resided in a spacious and sunny split-level house enclosed by high walls and a wrought-iron gate that opened and closed electronically. Her house had four bedrooms, two baths, a dining room, and a den that featured a television set and a stereo and shelves filled with books and record albums. The eat-in kitchen was equipped with the latest model refrigerator, gas range, and dishwasher. The utility room contained a washer and dryer. Family photographs crowded the mantelpiece over the fireplace in the living room, and the walls were hung with tasteful paintings and posters.

A big German shepherd and several fat cats wandered amiably about the property, which included a small but well-kept garden, a shimmering swimming pool, and separate maid's quarters in what had once been a garage. A brick courtyard provided ample parking space for two cars.

It was the home of Gail Johnson, her husband, their young daughter, and her teenage son. They were by no means wealthy, but they were comfortably affluent, solidly middle class, and, most important, upwardly mobile. Unlike Daphne and Cynthia and Ruth and their children, unlike everyone in the village where they then lived, the Johnsons could reach for more. They were free to expand their lives and improve them, quite at liberty to entertain aspirations and expectations, encouraged to plan and work toward a future that could be even more affluent and comfortable. Unlike Daphne, they could be certain that their reach need not always exceed their grasp.

Alan Johnson, the man of the house, was an immigrant. He had arrived from England in the early 1970s to assist in putting the country's first television station on the air. Until then, in those presatellite days, there had been no TV at all for South Africans. Condemned and forbidden by the apartheid government as a dangerous instrument of social and political corruption, it had finally been reluctantly approved, with the strict proviso that its content would be tightly controlled, its news broadcasts rigidly censored. With the experience and expertise he had gained from his work as a producer with the British Broadcasting Corporation, Alan had walked in on the ground floor of a golden opportunity. In almost no time at all, he had become—as he would put it—a "chap" of some importance at the SABC, the South African Broadcasting Corporation, a person of considerable value to the fledgling operation.

He was a stranger in a strange land, an alien resident of a foreign country, far from his roots. He was a man of above-average intelligence, to be sure, fairly well educated and quite hardworking—but in South Africa his most important credential was his color. Because Alan Johnson was white, all things were possible. By the mid-1980s he had left his job at SABC and with shrewd diligence had parlayed it and the connections it had offered into his own production company, providing sports coverage for the broadcasting outlet he'd helped establish and the others it was now spawning.

His wife had been similarly successful, though her success had been won at a much higher price. Without benefit of a college degree, Gail had managed nevertheless to carve out a niche for herself in Johannesburg's bustling and highly competitive business community, not a particularly cordial place for career women, even those who were native born. But from adolescence on, she had been ambitious and stubbornly self-sufficient. To her quick intelligence and her extraordinary stores of energy (she likened her metabolism to a hummingbird's), she added a nearly neurotic attention to detail and a veneer of toughness. She had toiled long and hard at a succession of respectable but modestly salaried jobs in banking and hotels, and now, like her husband, she had her own company, a small public-relations firm she had christened Gail Force.

An effervescent and sometimes bewildering blend of stark contrasts, she was hard-nosed yet softhearted, sharp-tongued yet congenitally kind, a marvelous friend but a malevolent enemy. She could be magnanimous. She could be petty. She was generous to a fault and passionately self-centered—and even in those days, she understood all this about herself. "I suppose it's safe to say that I was and am slightly complicated," she would reflect much later.

Yet, despite her complexities, she and Alan presented the very image of an ideal South African couple—for that matter, an ideal couple anywhere. To all appearances they were doting parents, merry partners, hard workers dedicated to their separate businesses and careers, yet committed to each other and to building a life together for themselves and their family. At least so it seemed to most of their friends, including those other middle-class couples the Johnsons had invited over for a New Year's Eve barbecue on the last evening of 1988.

It was also Alan's view. From his perspective, things could not have been much better. There was purple jacaranda in the garden, the water in the pool was heated, his company was expanding slowly, and his work was challenging and enjoyable. He regarded his little girl as a joy, he had firmly bonded with his wife's son, and most if not all of their friends were a pleasure. Not everything was perfect, of course, but there were compensating assets for almost every liability. If apartheid and the other racist politics and policies of his adopted country occasionally pricked his British conscience (England, after all, had been among the earliest of nations to outlaw slavery and to try to eliminate its practice), he comforted himself with the knowledge that he'd had nothing to do with devising and perpetuating them and was certainly in no position to do anything about them. No good purpose would have been served by any further exploration of that territory, he had long since decided. It was fair to say that he was reasonably pleased with the way things were going in his life.

For Gail it was a different story.

Like many progressive-minded and well-meaning whites in South Africa, she had long been horrified by the government's unyielding repression of black people. She had more or less agreed with her husband's assessment that there didn't seem to be any likely remedy, but for Gail, unlike him, that sense of futility seemed to eat at her, to gnaw at her conscience. She wanted desperately to do something, anything, but had no idea what role she could realistically play. She spoke of her angst with no one, including her husband. It was her secret, and keeping it hidden away as she did only made it grow in her mind.

For another thing, her little PR firm was in trouble. As long as the national economy had been humming along, Gail Force had done quite well. Its list of clients had grown and its monthly billings had increased, but when the economy slowed even slightly, the public-relations sector was among the first to feel the pinch—and with international sanctions punishing South Africa for its racist policies, it had become more and more difficult for Gail to keep the firm's head above water, much less post a half-decent profit. Each month she was working harder and longer for less money. She had already let one employee go and was seriously considering further reductions of her small staff; at home she was trying to decide whether she should or could dismiss the family's longtime maid as well.

Yet, as important as her business was to her—and indeed it had become one of the pillars of her life, both in terms of the income it supplied her household and for the immense pride she derived from having built it from nothing—what was also gnawing at her on the final evening of 1988 was her marriage. Whatever Alan's evaluation may have been (she wasn't too certain, since he generally avoided all talk about "the relationship"), to her it seemed completely devoid of energy and passion. She saw it as a dead fish, floating cold in the stagnant matrimonial waters. The marriage had always been a bit fractious, but she had managed to rationalize that as simply an inevitable by-product of her naturally combative personality and the brusque, take-no-prisoners, in-your-face style that she believed was the key to her survival in the world of business.

"If I thought something was worth an argument, however trivial it might have seemed to others, I damn well argued," she would later say. Alan, determined to avoid confrontation with her, would go to great lengths to stay uninvolved—but sooner or later, usually as a result of her relentless goading, he would be drawn in. "And eventually," Gail recalled, "whatever it was, we would settle it or maybe we wouldn't—but at least we cared enough to raise our voices."

For some time, however, even that had been missing. There had been few arguments. Alan had learned how to step aside, to leave the ring without a fight. In her view, without the old energizing conflicts, the spats that as often as not ended with passionate reconciliations in bed, their marriage had fallen mute. "It was driving me bonkers," she said. "I think, looking back now, that I was quite honestly going mad." She did not dislike Alan—not then, at least and in fact often enjoyed his company. In his mid-forties by then, he was a physically attractive fellow, tall and rather lean, with only a hint of middle-aged paunch beginning to show. If he sometimes seemed distant and detached, he could also be quite affable and genuinely funny. Gail knew him to be essentially a kind and generous man who had made a sincere effort to reach out to her son. Still, although she suspected him (without a shred of evidence) of having an affair, she declined to accuse him, not because she didn't dare but because she didn't care. In fact, she was casually looking to have one herself.

She could see no promising candidates for a romantic fling among the men who were in the group celebrating New Year's Eve at their home on the evening of December 31, 1988. They were all discussing sports, their jobs, their children, and occasionally drifting cautiously into the realm of politics, including the transfer of Nelson Mandela to a more comfortable minimum-security facility, which was just about the extent of their knowledge of his new status. They had no real confidence that anything would come of it. After all, President Botha had insisted on Mandela's "cooperation" as a requirement for his release, which meant Mandela would have to renounce and condemn violence as a means of change in the country. Surely the old man would never consent to that. Still, even the merest possibility of Mandela's freedom had given politics a new dimension. Essentially, though, the men around the Johnsons' pool that night were like Daphne and her family: They paid very little attention to such matters. Mandela had been in jail since before most of them were born—certainly since before Alan had come to South Africa—and they more or less assumed that was probably where he would die.

None of the men or their wives regarded themselves as racists. They believed that the bigotry for which their country had by then become internationally notorious was the foul product of the Afrikaners who had run the country for the last forty years. Although the group that had assembled in Gail's home considered themselves to be as South African as the Afrikaners, their own roots were mainly English, which most of them believed to be a gene pool clearly superior to the Afrikaners'. They would admit that they were a part of the system and profited from its built-in preference for whites, but they could see no way to change it. Mainly they went about their lives persuading themselves that while the status quo was objectionable, it was also beyond alteration. For Gail their passionless passivity, especially Alan's, was grating.

"I know I'm very high-maintenance," she would conclude, "but here was this guy, my husband, always sitting on the sidelines, usually on the couch, always miles away, usually ignoring me, ignoring the news, ignoring all the realities of living in Johannesburg and in South Africa, ignoring everything except sports, not caring much about anything I cared about, except the children maybe, reading his goddamn newspaper, looking for the British football results. I was enraged by that, enraged by his inability or his unwillingness to make real contact with me or with the things I considered really important."

Like South Africa itself, Gail and Alan had reached a crisis point, and as Gail passed the hors d'oeuvres on that New

Year's Eve, navigating through the small talk and the cocktail chatter of her guests, she experienced an epiphany of sorts. As though from a great height, she looked down on herself standing on the patio beside the pool and saw her own image, not in realistic human form but as an indistinct line drawing, minus any distinguishing features. It was *her* outline, but it was incomplete, blank, empty.

Suddenly it occurred to her that night that she desperately wanted—no, absolutely *required*—something more, or at least something other, than this life. Not a bigger house in a better neighborhood, and not a more expensive car or a more stylish wardrobe or a larger bank account for herself or her business or her family. That much she understood.

Later that evening, as 1988 faded into the past and glasses clinked with toasts to the future, to each other, and to their mutual good fortune in the coming year, she found herself standing slightly apart from the fun and the traditional festivities, silent and sad.

Mary Gail Johnson was forty years old. "Is this it?" she asked herself that night. "Is this really all there is?" It wasn't.

S everal years before, in another neighborhood of Johannesburg, I had been introduced to the Reverend Dr. Beyers Naude, one of South Africa's most remarkable citizens. Once a respected clergyman and leading voice in the Dutch Reformed Church (the Afrikaners' traditional faith), he was the son of one of South Africa's most distinguished Afrikaner families. His father had been a founding member of the influential

all-male society called the Broederbond—"the brotherhood"—
which would eventually count among its members many of
the most powerful in the country's elite Afrikaner hierarchy.
For those in government and law, in medicine and the church,
in academia and in the military, belonging to the Broederbond
was a mark of achievement and trust within South Africa's
inner circles. Like his father, Beyers Naude had grown up
within a world made snug and comfortable by shared connections and convictions.

By the mid-1970s, however, along with a few other prominent whites—few enough that they might all have comfortably convened in his living room—Dr. Naude had summarily
rejected apartheid, publicly, from the pulpit of the same
church that had served as the soil from which the country's
racism had sprouted and grown. In an eloquent homily one
morning, he had condemned apartheid as unchristian, as sinful
and immoral. For his courage, the eminent clergyman incurred the wrath of his fellow Afrikaners, both within and beyond his church. The government officially banned him from
making any public comments: no delivering sermons to any
congregation or writing articles for any publication or speaking with reporters or so much as participating in any conversation that included more than one other person. His phone
was tapped and his movements restricted, and because he was
suspected of having had some surreptitious communications
with Nelson Mandela in prison—which was true, and which
he freely admitted—he was kept under the constant surveil-
lance of security agents. Along with Helen Suzman and Nadine Gordimer, he was one of the South Africans I had sought

out and spoken with in reporting the story of antiapartheid whites. Years later, when I heard the news of Mandela's release and the jubilant celebrations in the streets, my first thought was of Dr. Naude and something he had told me that day in his living room.

In his mellifluous voice, heavily steeped in the odd accent of an Afrikaner's English, he said, "There is a miracle at work in this country. I use that term without any qualification whatsoever. It is a genuine miracle, I think, because otherwise, without some form of divine intervention in our affairs here, it would not and could not exist—and the miracle is this: Despite everything that has been done to the black people in this country, despite the generations of abuse and cruelty they have suffered at the hands of the white people of this country—despite all that, there remains within their collective heart an enormous reservoir of goodwill for the whites, for the very people who have perpetuated the system that has abused them for so long, that has enslaved them and disenfranchised them for all these years.

"Instead of anger and hatred and rancor and malice and an urge for vengeance—all of which would be completely understandable, if not completely justifiable—there is in their hearts a substantial deposit of affection and respect. It is on that foundation and that foundation alone—and not on the willingness of whites to change their views and their laws— that a new South Africa will be built. And it's my sincere belief that without that, there will never be a new South Africa."

I asked how much longer it could last, this reservoir of

goodwill, how much longer black South Africans could endure the daily denial of even the most basic of human rights without an explosion of rage and retribution.

"I don't know," Dr. Naude said.

He paused as he considered his answer, absentmindedly forming a steeple with his enormous hands and long fingers. "And I don't think anyone really knows. I must say that this is the greatest of my worries. Can it be quantified, this reservoir? How much *is* there, or how much *was* there, and how much of it is left? How much time do we have before it's depleted—and what will happen to the country when or if it's gone? That dwells on my mind throughout every single day I live, and it is in my prayers every night. My prayer is that the miracle will continue, that the well will prove to be bottomless, or, if not, then at least that the supply of grace and kindness and goodwill among blacks is sufficient to last until a new country can come into being."

In the genteel neighborhood where he had lived for years, his house was nearly silent. Beyond his well-kept lawn and across the street that ran in front of it, several white policemen lolled around their cars, keeping an eye on this fellow who was assumed to pose such a serious threat to the security of his country, simply because he had come to believe that all South Africans, regardless of race, were entitled to the basic rights afforded to all white South Africans—and because he had said so out loud.

Dr. Naude grew solemn. "Because, let me tell you as someone who knows both blacks and whites, if the miracle expires, if the well does run dry, then I believe there will be blood in the streets of South Africa—and the violence we have already seen here in days and years past will seem, in comparison, like a Sunday picnic."

In 1989, Gail Johnson was no more sensitive than anyone else to the emerging AIDS catastrophe in her country. Like most everyone she knew, she had no idea that women like Daphne and Thandie were passing it along to their babies. For Gail, as for a vast majority of the international medical community, AIDS still remained a disease of homosexual men— and even that fact she grasped only dimly. She had a vague understanding that some shadowy plague was operating in the gay community, but in 1989 she was neither curious nor concerned enough to expand on her minimal knowledge. She knew no one who was infected, and the only gays she knew were her sister and her companion.

Increasingly, Gail's energies were now focused on the daily struggle to keep her public-relations company alive in a dismal economy. South Africa's image in the outside world was already badly tainted, and it was growing worse. One of the most popular American films that year, *Lethal Weapon 2,* made much of its villains' South African accents. A growing number of American banks and corporations had adopted formal anti-apartheid codes, refusing to do any business or make any investments in South Africa. Many other companies and several countries had chosen to ignore the international sanctions and still bought and sold under the table, but the chief beneficiaries of such duplicity were the larger, well-connected businesses in the country, not struggling little enterprises like Gail's. She knew nothing of their subterfuge or how it worked; she knew only how nearly impossible it had become to remain solvent from one week to the next. New clients were rare, and old ones were declining to renew their contracts for her services. Still, she refused to surrender to what seemed to be the inevitable, not while hard work still held out the promise of at least the possibility of survival. So she worked harder and longer than ever before.

She could not bring that same commitment to her troubled marriage. With each day that passed, Gail seemed to be moving further away from her husband and becoming less concerned about the distance. Alan seemed to be separating himself from her as well. As with most dysfunctional couples, they were both trying very hard to minimize the effect of their estrangement on the children, going to great lengths to pretend for their benefit that nothing was wrong. Although the tension between them was nearly palpable, shouting was rare. Their mutual weapon of choice was silence.

In a sense Gail and Alan were not unlike the country in which they lived, for in 1989 what was undeniably true about South Africa was always unfailingly denied. It is not a perfect analogy, of course. The black and white people who lived there were not married, but they were all residents of the same house, so to speak—and plainly their incompatibility was fast approaching a point of no return. South Africa simply could not continue to exist as a nation while systematically denying the rights or in some cases the very existence of 40 million of its citizens, thousands of whom were increasingly willing to protest against its inequities peacefully but also, if finally necessary, to violently dismantle the country as a means of freeing themselves from the shackles of apartheid. The government and de Klerk, its new leader, were still committed to preserving as much of the old South Africa as possible, the one in which most of its white population had richly prospered for so long, even going to such lengths as encouraging factional warfare within the black community in an attempt to weaken its resolve. For quite some time, South Africa's security forces had been training and arming black paramilitary groups, predominantly Zulus, and encouraging them to attack other blacks who expressed opposition to the government. The logic was fairly simple: The more blacks who were fighting each other, the fewer there would be to stand against the government. In January 1990 alone, more than a hundred people, all of them black, were killed as a result of such internecine violence.

There were also state-sanctioned death squads on the prowl in the country, murdering antiapartheid leaders and other activists. In Cape Town a white neo-Nazi rally went unmolested by police while Bishop Desmond Tutu, the Nobel Peace laureate, and other clergymen were arrested for staging a counter-demonstration—and Tutu's new organization, the Committee for the Defense of Decency, formed to fill the vacuum after several other black groups had been outlawed, was itself banned by the government. In frustration, and in a striking departure from his previous position, Tutu stated publicly that for black South Africans seeking justice, there seemed to be no alternative but violence. On both sides of the great chasm, the violence continued and escalated.

In those days, the country "was a wreck, a total wreck," Gail remembered. "There were all sorts of rumors. There was talk that Mandela would be released, there was talk that he would never be released. No one knew what to believe, and, to tell the truth, very few people believed anything at all until it actually happened."

If it had achieved little else, the Afrikaners' government had managed to plant the seeds of fear among whites—fear of racial massacres, fear of retribution killings, fear of widespread unrest and rioting, fear of blood in the streets—if blacks should ever obtain true personal and political freedom. Even Gail, who abhorred apartheid, was not immune to such anxieties. She knew and had worked with many black people, and many had worked for her. She had always respected them as individuals, she said, and had always treated them as such. She greatly admired many of those she knew personally, admired them for their courage, for the hardships they endured to take care of those they loved. The possibility that they would perhaps be united someday in a single political force did not worry her. What did cross her mind, however, was that if South Africa did not change, and soon, they might very well be united in a single force of violence. "God knows, they had reasons to seek revenge," she said.

Still, when Nelson Mandela was released in February 1990—just a few days after Xolani Nkosi's first birthday—it was a moment of exhilaration for Gail, a moment of great joy and enormous relief. It seemed to be a sign that history was finally being taken in a new direction, that it had veered off the path so familiar to her and to others in South Africa and was headed toward some exciting uncharted territory. Gail saw Mandela's release as a promise, or at least as an opportunity. After a lifetime of standing outside the mainstream of her community and her culture, perhaps she, too, might find a place at last where she could feel she belonged.

The day Mandela's freedom was granted, Gail quietly celebrated his new status, pouring a glass of wine for her maid and for herself. Together the two women toasted their future in a *new* South Africa. Years later, Gail would vividly remember that day. "It really seemed to me as though he was not the only one getting out of prison," she said. "It was like some huge door was swinging open for all the rest of us, too, for everybody in the country, for all the whites and blacks and coloreds, and we could all walk through it—together. You cannot imagine how much I hated the way it had always been, and yet I could not imagine then how I could be a part of what it could become."

She would be gravely disappointed when many thousands of her fellow whites, both Afrikaners and Anglos, would choose not to walk through that metaphorical door, and it would be some time before even the dimmest vision of a new country was realized. Still, on that February afternoon in 1989, Gail knew that it had finally begun.

If Gail saw herself as an outsider, it was not merely because her views on race cut against the grain in white South Africa. In fact, from the time she was a little girl, she had felt that she did not belong—did not belong in her family, did not belong in the towns and cities where she lived, did not belong at the boarding schools she attended.

"I just understood that that was the way it was for me," she would say later, a trace of melancholy in her voice. "I understand now that it might not have been true, not really, but even if it wasn't, I believed it to be true, and believed it long enough and passionately enough that it eventually became something akin to my religion. I just did not belong."

Like Daphne's mother, Ruth Khumalo, Gail was born almost precisely at the onset of the Afrikaners' disastrous grip on government power. That was in July 1948, in a hospital in Port Elizabeth, a city on the Indian Ocean known to most South Africans as PE—to an elementary-school teacher in her mid-twenties, an attractive and well-educated woman from a respectable family, conscientious about her work and devoted to the children in her classroom. But she was also a single woman who, for one reason or another, could not or would not marry the father of her child. In those days, in the white communities of South Africa—in stark contrast to the Zulu culture in which Ruth and Daphne had grown up—there was a serious social penalty to be paid for being pregnant without being married. After considerable and no doubt painful deliberation, Gail's mother chose not to suffer the inevitable alienation of her family and the certain opprobrium of her community. She could not see how she could manage raising a child by herself, alone and without a husband and father.

"I don't really know, but I think I was quite possibly the product of a one-night stand," Gail said. "It's nothing to be ashamed of—I've never been in the least ashamed of it—because it's just one of those things that happens when your body takes over from your brain. Believe me, I know about that. It can happen to anybody and, in this particular case, it probably happened to my mother."

Gail's mother had already made arrangements through the hospital for her adoption (abortions were illegal, and people willing to perform them were few and far between), and in the first week of her life, the baby was transferred to a local orphanage. Two or three weeks later, she officially became Mary Gail, the daughter of Jeff and Jessie Roberts, a bank executive and his wife—both Anglos with English roots, not Afrikaners. She was taken, bundled against the cold, to their comfortable middle-class home in Cradock, a quaint little frontier town in the middle of a wilderness a hundred miles or so north of Port Elizabeth.

Gail's new parents had also adopted another little girl three years before. They were a doting couple, pleased beyond reason to have children of their own, including this

most recent addition, a dark-haired daughter with large, ex-
pressive eyes. Jeff and Jessie Roberts were devoted to both
their children, Mary Gail and her older sister, Colleen. Neither would want for anything

Colleen had come to them in much the same circumstances as Gail had. A single woman, pregnant by some fellow
to whom marriage was not a reasonable alternative, had been
willing to surrender her baby to a couple eager to have her. As
the two girls grew older, neighbors and friends inevitably
began offering the comments so often made about adopted
children: how uncanny it was that they physically resembled
one or both of their adoptive parents, or how much the
girls—the sisters who shared no genes—even seemed to look
a bit like each other.

"Which was ludicrous, of course," Gail would say. "Colleen
and I did not in the least resemble each other, nor did either
one of us bear the slightest resemblance to our parents. But
that's the way it was. Everybody wanted to put the best possible face on everything. I suppose they were being kind."

Jessie Roberts was a housewife, and her husband was employed as an executive at the South African Land Bank, a national institution established to provide loans to the country's
farmers. They lived comfortably on his modest salary, but they
would never be wealthy.

"He didn't own the bank, of course," Gail said of Jeff
Roberts. "He may have been an officer in it, but I'm not really
sure. People respected him and treated him well, and they
treated us well, too. After all, he was the fellow who approved
their loans. Basically, though, I think he was just an appa-

ratchik, more than a clerk but still just a working stiff who
happened to wear a suit and tie to his job and sit behind a
desk."

Though not of his own choosing, he was something of a
nomad, subject to a series of transfers that uprooted him and
his family several times during Gail's childhood and adolescence. The first move was from Cradock to Bloemfontein,
where they lived until Gail was about five years old.

The next transfer took them to Beaufort West. There,
when Gail was six or seven years old, Jessie Roberts sat her
down in the parlor of their house for the obligatory mother-
to-daughter discussion of the birds and the bees, "about which
she knew next to nothing herself," Gail said.

In later years Gail would realize that it seemed fairly early
in her life to be discussing such matters, but she remembers
the occasion most for something else. It was also then that
Mrs. Roberts revealed to Gail that both she and Colleen had
been adopted.

"I remember exactly what she said," Gail declared.

"First she said that all babies come out of their mothers'
tummies. Then she said that, unlike our little friends, who had
all come out of their mothers' tummies, we hadn't come out
of hers. Then she said that made us very special children, because she and Jeff had personally chosen us. We were special
kids, she said, 'because we picked you out.'"

Gail asked her why she had been chosen.

"Because," said Mrs. Roberts, "of your big brown eyes."

Gail nodded.

"And also because you had little pimples on your fanny."

Gail would later say that she had been much more curious about the condition of her derriere as an infant than with the fact that she had been adopted.

She asked no further questions.

Her recollections of that day are among the kinder memories she has retained of the woman who had become her mother. As Gail grew older, their relationship became increasingly strained.

By the time Gail entered early adolescence, Jeff Roberts had been promoted and transferred several times. For Gail, however, one home was as unpleasant as the last. She saw them all as places where conformity was elevated to a virtue, where nothing mattered so much as the veneer of respectability, where propriety outranked reality, for her parents and for everyone else in the community. Almost as soon as she learned what "hypocrisy" meant, it became one of her favorite words.

"My parents were not overtly racist in their attitudes or their behavior," she said. "I mean by that that they didn't speak badly of black people and didn't abuse those who worked for them at the bank or in our house. But they could hardly help being a product of their time and their place."

When Gail was eleven, the family moved from Beaufort West to Potchefstroom, a little city in northwestern South Africa, once the capital of the Afrikaners' first republic. She was enrolled in a prestigious all-girls school she came to hate for its rigid rules and regulations.

Seen as something of a problem, Gail was often in trouble and quite unhappy there most of the time. Nonetheless, when her father was again promoted and transferred to another branch of the bank in Pietersburg, her parents decided that, however miserable she might have been, she would remain behind in Potchefstroom as a boarder at the school. Until then, despite her dissatisfaction, her grades had been average or better. After her parents left, however, her academic performance began to deteriorate. The appropriate letters were sent to her parents, informing them of their daughter's alarming lack of progress.

"The only time we were allowed off the premises of the school was on Sunday to walk in single-file to church," she recalled. "Saturday nights we used to have 'dancing' in the school hall. No boys, mind you. We danced with each other. If that's not promoting lesbianism, then I don't know what is—and if I ever hear 'Soldier Boy' again in my life, I'll scream."

By the time she was in the ninth grade, she had come to regard the school in Potchefstroom as a virtual prison. She repeatedly wrote to her parents, pleading with them to arrange a transfer—and they finally agreed. She joined them in Pietersburg and entered Capricorn High School, but when her father was transferred yet again, she remained behind again as a boarder. Nevertheless, she seemed to prosper and was made a prefect (a student leader) before she lost her rank when she was caught smoking. When she graduated, she rejoined her family in Pietermaritzburg. It was far from a joyous reunion. She found their household to be as stale and stilted as she had remembered it in all the other places.

Almost at once, she and her mother were in serious conflict, at odds over almost everything—from the way Gail preferred to dress to her language, from her choice of friends and

the company she kept, especially the young men, to her flout-
ing of a nightly curfew.

Gail, about to turn eighteen, was probably no more rebel-
lious than millions of other teenagers. Similarly, Jessie Roberts was no more inept than millions of frustrated mothers.
Still, the effect of their steady conflict was erosive. Little by
little, it ate away at whatever bonds may have existed between
them until, at last, each retreated into a cold silence that would
characterize their relationship for years to come.

Pietermaritzburg is a city steeped—or embalmed, as Gail
would say—in the Boer mythology, the Afrikaner legend.
Founded in 1838 on the edge of the Zulus' beloved Valley of a
Thousand Hills, it is dominated by the Victorian architecture
of its early days. Moreover, it is an altar at which Afrikaners
worship their history. Included in the standard tour of the city
is the imposing Church of the Vow, built to memorialize the
Battle of Blood River, in which white settlers who had mi-
grated out to the region had slaughtered hundreds of Zulus,
who were unhappy with their presence. The city was named
for Pieter Retief and Gert Maritz, both important Afrikaner
icons, and has served as the capital first of Natalia and then of
Natal. Its striking parliament building, with impressive col-
umns and bright copper domes, stands as a relic of the city's
golden age, which lasted for more than a century, when the
population swelled from an influx of Germans and British.
The Germans were warmly welcomed by the Afrikaners; the
British, including Gail's parents, were still suspect years after
the wars. For many of the Afrikaners in Pietermaritzburg the
only saving grace of the British was that they were not black.

As Gail struggled with her problems as a teenager trying to become a woman, she was not unaware of the history of the place. It was where Mohandas Gandhi was unceremoniously evicted from a train one night after refusing to surrender his seat on an all-white coach; the place where, in the nocturnal chill of the deserted railroad station, Gandhi had meditated until dawn and decided to remain in South Africa to fight its racism. Samuel Langhorne Clemens, better known as Mark Twain, had visited Pietermaritzburg, and a grand funeral procession for Prince Imperial Louis Napoleon had wound its way through the streets in 1879 after he was slain by Zulus. And while it wasn't on the tourist maps or recorded in the city's official chronicles, other, more recent history occurred there as well. Nelson Mandela, as a fledgling attorney, had made his first appearance in a South African courtroom there (and, years later, his last speech as president of the country), and only a few miles away, in the tiny town of Harwich—not far from the settlement where Ruth Khumalo and her family had lived—Mandela's arrest in 1962 had marked the beginning of his long incarceration.

Jeff and Jessie Roberts loved the city. "It wasn't the racism— the apartheid—that was so built into the place," Gail later said. "That wasn't what appealed to them. It was just the order of it, all the neatly organized predictability. That's why they liked it, I think. Everybody had a place. Everybody had a status."

Gail's sister, Colleen, was less dramatic in her rejection of the lifestyle and values in Pietermaritzburg and in her adoptive parents' home. She was more conciliatory to them, but no less determined to go her own way. Not long after Gail arrived, following her high school graduation, Colleen moved out, headed for Johannesburg. Her departure was upsetting for Gail. Despite the three-year difference in their ages, they had grown quite close. Now Gail felt even more alone.

Her father arranged a clerk's job for her at a local bank, but she soon had enough of it, and enough of living at home with her parents. Casting about for new opportunities, she landed an entry-level job at one of the luxury hotels in Victoria Falls, on the Zambezi River, far from Pietermaritzburg, on the border between Zambia and what was then Rhodesia. When she boarded the bus for Johannesburg, headed for Victoria Falls, she did not look back. She was nearly twenty years old. "I wanted to make my own mistakes," she said. She would.

Victoria Falls is one of southern Africa's truly grand experiences. All the power of the continent seems to gather itself into the surging Zambezi as it roars toward a thunderously spectacular cataract. The noise is deafening, the mist rising from the rocks below constantly thick in the air. In this natural wonderland, free of any restrictions for the first time in her young life, Gail was as close to being happy as she would ever be for years to come. She worked as both clerk and greeter, welcoming guests at the door with some snappy patter about the joyous time they were about to have. She had been assigned a room in the staff dormitory and reveled in her freedom to do as she pleased during her nonworking hours, which eventually included a torrid romance with one of the other hotel employees.

"Devilishly handsome," she said of him years later. "Tall and dark and—I thought at the time—suave and sophisticated.

Maybe he was, maybe he wasn't. I don't know, but I do know I did see him as Cary Grant, and I thought I was Audrey Hepburn or Grace Kelly."

Soon, however, the Hollywood fantasy was punctured: She was pregnant. The young man was surprised to hear her news. He was uninterested in a future together as parents, and he made it clear that he considered her condition to be *her* problem.

There was no thought of an abortion. They were illegal, of course, not only in Zambia, where she was working, but also back in South Africa. Still, legal or not, they were available in both countries, but it was an alternative Gail simply didn't consider. "It might have been a solution for some girls back then, and it might be a solution for some girls now, but it just never occurred to me. If it wasn't *his* problem, then it wasn't *his* baby. It was mine, and I was going to have it."

The romance ended as soon as she told the young man. After a few months, when her pregnancy began to be obvious, Gail contacted her sister in Johannesburg. Colleen was wonderfully supportive, and nonjudgmental, no doubt in part because she knew what it was to defy social norms. Now openly gay, she was living happily with her partner.

When Gail arrived in Johannesburg, she stayed with Colleen for a while before checking in at what was euphemistically known in those days as a "home for wayward women." Colleen assured her that she would be well cared for and that she would not have to decide about giving up the baby for adoption, if that turned out to be her choice, until after its birth.

Eventually Gail's adoptive parents were told. When the time seemed right, Jeff and Jessie drove to Johannesburg. Her father was typically noncommittal, but her mother urged her not to keep the baby she was carrying—to give the nuns permission to arrange for its adoption, then to return to Pietermaritzburg, to the forgiving embrace of her family. Gail did not feel that she needed to be forgiven, and she was not at all interested in going back to a home she'd hated in the first place. "I don't know if I would have rejected adoption if my mother had not so strongly endorsed it," she later said, "but I could not at that point imagine going back into that house, with or without my baby."

Jessie tried repeatedly, both before and after the baby's birth in January 1970, to persuade Gail not to keep it, but Gail was absolutely adamant, and Colleen supported her. After seeing their new grandson one time, Gail's parents left for the long drive home. Like millions of parents all over the world, they were no doubt wondering where they had gone wrong, asking themselves how two girls raised in what they had intended to be a loving and wholesome home, given every opportunity to be as successful and as happy as they themselves had been, had somehow managed to stray so far from the path of their own example.

So Gail and her new son moved in with her sister and her companion. She soon found another job in another hotel, one of the best in Johannesburg, where one day a television producer from England checked in. Alan Johnson had suddenly become a part of her life.

Alan seemed impressively smart and capable, as well as quite
worldly and sophisticated. If he also at times seemed emotionally bottled up and quite restained—"so damned British"—
Gail was a single woman with an illegitimate child, after all,
and she knew that the odds were overwhelmingly against
her. So, after physical intimacy led to something deeper and
he proposed to her, she resolved to make a go of it as *Mrs.
Alan Johnson*. Her parents were delighted. They visited often
now—more often than Gail liked, at least—and generously
provided the funds that allowed the new couple to purchase a
house in a pleasant Johannesburg neighborhood. Before long,
after a difficult pregnancy, their only child together was born
in 1981, a little girl they named Nicolette.

FOUR

And so Gail and Alan settled into their lives together, into the stable, if not idyllic, rhythm that by decade's end would seem increasingly suffocating. Change was inevitable, but Gail had no idea when or from where it would come.

As it happened, it came on a morning a few months after Mandela's release in early 1990, when she took a call in her office from her old friend Carol. Both had been students at Potchefstroom but, over the years, had lost track of each other. They had met again in Johannesburg, renewed their friendship, and had seen each other with some frequency ever since.

On their way to a restaurant, Carol asked if Gail minded a bit of a detour and a slight delay. She said she wanted to stop by and see her older brother, who was alone in his apartment and not feeling well. She had a few groceries for him, and some magazines and books as well. Gail happily agreed. What were a few minutes more or less?

In fact, Carol's brother was in the terminal stages of AIDS. "I was stunned by his appearance," Gail later said. "I had never seen anything like it before. He was almost, quite literally, skin and bones. He was in bed and could barely move, could hardly speak at all, nothing above a whisper—and there he was, all alone in this dingy, dark apartment. It was like a dungeon. The disease was his death sentence, and he was there in his prison cell, awaiting execution. That's what it seemed like to me. I must say I was shocked, and for one of the few times in my life, I was speechless."

The two women bathed him, prepared a light meal for him, fed him, and sat with him for quite some time. Gail read to him from one of the magazines Carol had brought along. Their own lunch was forgotten. Afterward, when they left the apartment, Carol told Gail that her family had rejected her brother because of his homosexuality. They had informed him that he was not welcome in their home ever again, and had not visited him at all since he'd fallen ill.

"So who looks after him?" Gail asked.

"Just me," said Carol. "When I can."

"Does he have any friends? Isn't there somebody else?"

"I'm afraid it's just me," said Carol.

Outside Gail's office they sat in the car, held hands, and wept.

"But," Gail said later, "I knew there was much more to do than just sit and cry into our Kleenex. What I saw there that day in that awful apartment—that man alone, dying alone, with no one to talk to, no one to smile at him, no one to touch him or show him that he was not alone—what I saw there that day was for me just intolerable. Simply unacceptable." That evening, at home, she made an effort to tell Alan, her husband, about her experience but found herself unable to articulate exactly what had taken place and how she had responded to it. "Never, never in my life had I seen anything like that," she said. "I had no words to describe it, not to Alan, not to anybody else. I was traumatized by it."

But her trauma energized her. She was determined to do something. She began by spending hours researching AIDS and finding out as much as she could about its incidence in Johannesburg's homosexual community. In those days gay men in South Africa, as in many other cultures around the world, were generally in the closet, keeping their lifestyles and sexual preference a secret. There were a few exceptions, of course—men who had come to terms with their sexuality and did not concern themselves with whether anyone else approved—but such exceptions were still rare. Nevertheless, male homosexuality, as Gail soon discovered, was also a fact of life in every facet of the population. Hidden away as shameful or at least unacceptable in respectable circles, it was still common among whites, blacks, and people of mixed racial backgrounds. It cut across most of the demographic strata. There were gay men among the educated and among the illiterate, among the rich and the poor and the middle class.

Similarly, AIDS was not restricted by apartheid in its array of victims.

In the early 1990s, in contrast to much of the rest of Africa, where most of the black population lived, in South Africa AIDS had not yet become a threat to white women or their children. In the white community, it still remained a men's disease—and, more specifically, a disease of *gay* men. In fact, studies point squarely to a South African Airways flight attendant—a gay white man—as the carrier for the first infectious transfer of the virus from Africa to North America.

For Gail, however, it was not a matter of statistics or demographics or epidemiology. For her the point was the haunting image of Carol's brother dying alone in his apartment. "I knew I could do nothing about the disease itself, and I knew I didn't know enough about it to become much of an educator on the subject—not just then, at any rate—so I concentrated on how alienated and alone those who had AIDS usually were. That was the most important thing I found out—that people with AIDS were cut off from everybody and everything. I believed there was some way to help them. That's what I was searching for."

Her search included consultations with business associates, with those in the public-relations sector of Johannesburg, with her husband's colleagues in the television business, with their friends and their neighbors. She badgered them for any information they might have about the disease: What did they know about it? Did they know anyone who was infected? What was being done to help them? She talked with dozens of doctors and lawyers. She met a prominent judge who was gay. Gradually she assembled a small network of people, both gay and heterosexual, and in the process discovered that there were other South Africans as concerned as she was about AIDS and its effects on those who had it. By October 1990, a small group of them had raised enough money among themselves to lease and furnish an old mansion in Houghton, one of the city's more prestigious neighborhoods, to which they welcomed a dozen or so residents who had at least two things in common: They were all gay, and they were all dying of AIDS.

As 1991 approached, Gail Johnson was forty-two years old. Her marriage was not improving, it's true, but otherwise her sense of detachment from her own life was beginning to fade. At the old mansion in Houghton, among the dying men, in the company of others who cared as much about them as she did, she found a place where she thought, just maybe, she might belong. It was called the Guest House.

In the well-manicured surroundings of Houghton, the Guest House became a comfortable refuge for its dozen or so residents. Not all the neighbors were pleased to have a gathering of gay men just next door or across the tree-lined street, but only a few complained, and none very loudly or with much insistence.

It was half haven and half hospice. It not only fed and housed the men but also provided a steady stream of companionship for them—various volunteers from her expanding network who would stop by on their way to their jobs or on their way home or over the weekend, spending an hour or so chatting with them, reading to the men, watching television or playing cards or board games, preparing and serving food, cleaning the bedrooms and the baths. Eventually even some of the neighbors began dropping by to help.

When he could find the time, Gail's son, Brett, also worked on the informal staff. Brett had just turned twenty-one the previous January and was serving in the South African military as a marine. Responding to his service notice had been a difficult decision for him. A few young men had refused, but then they faced either leaving the country illegally or going to jail. Gail had told Brett she would support whatever choice he made. He did not want to leave his family and sneak away, and so he had decided on what he believed was the lesser of two evils. He had no confidence in either the integrity or the future of the government, but he refused to abandon his country. A tall, strapping fellow with his mother's large, dark eyes, he would often come home on a weekend pass, hang his uniform in the closet of his old bedroom, don civilian clothes, and head for the Guest House.

Alan did his share as well, even organized a couple of fundraising events; and their ten-year-old daughter, Nicolette, was also a regular, puttering about and pretending to dust and clean but usually watching television with the residents. All in all, the place was working, accomplishing what those who had created it had intended. It was clean and safe, warm in the mild winter, shaded and cool in the summer, and the dying men were never alone. Not only did they have each other, they had a circle of genuine friends in their lives. The Guest House was a success.

"Except for money," Gail said. "That was always a big problem. The residents who could pay a little did, but there was just never enough—not for food, not for the rent, not for repairs or maintenance, not for gas for vans to take the men to their doctors or to the hospital. It was tough. We were just scrimping and scraping along from one week to the next. We had our little fund-raisers and subscription drives, of course, but they never produced much. We never knew how long it would be possible to keep it going."

Somehow they did—mostly by digging into their own pockets every week to make up the difference. As time passed, word of the place began to spread throughout the city and even out into the black townships. There were two or three stories about it in the local newspapers and even a short television feature on an SABC evening newscast.

By late May even Daphne had heard about the Guest House from the doctor who was treating Xolani. The doctor had recently confirmed her worst fears: Her son was also infected with the AIDS virus.

Daphne was deeply despondent by then, Cynthia recalled, trying desperately to keep the family going, working at odd jobs around Benoni and Daveyton, taking the boy back and forth to the hospital for more tests and treatment, struggling to cope with the devastating truth that it was she who had infected him. Cynthia thought Daphne began to see herself as a daughter who could not take care of her mother, as an older sister who could not look after a younger one, and as a mother who believed that not only was she failing both her children but that she had poisoned her baby son.

Moreover, Daphne had become anxious about the increasing level of hostility toward her and the boy from some of their new neighbors in the little squatters' camp, many of whom seemed to subscribe to the same notions about AIDS as had her former employer and her former landlady. Even Ruth, her own mother, seemed less and less interested in keeping the family together. She and the neighbors were frightened of the mysterious disease and those who were infected with it. Some of the neighbors had made veiled threats. Others were not so subtle. One day Daphne found a menacing note left under a stone in the dirt in front of their shanty. It said simply *Leave!*

When she read it, she made a radical decision.

In the first week of June 1991—the beginning of South Africa's autumn—with her little boy in tow, she headed out from the squatters' camp into Daveyton. From there she found her way into Johannesburg, and finally to Houghton and the Guest House. She climbed the broad stairs that led up from the wide lawn and knocked on the large, imposing door.

It was opened by Warrick Allen, the acting director of the hospice. He introduced himself and asked Daphne to come in. Noticing her weariness, he invited her to sit down in the living room, disappeared into the kitchen, and returned with a cup of tea.

"Now, what can we do for you?" he asked, handing her the steaming cup.

Daphne's English was not polished, but with neither preliminaries nor small talk she managed to make it clear to Allen that she wanted her little boy to live in the Guest House. She explained that she had AIDS and he was also infected, that she knew she would soon be unable to take care of him, and that people were saying bad things about them where they lived. She seemed on the verge of tears.

"Can he come and stay in this place?" Daphne asked.

Allen told her he could not give her an immediate answer but asked her to wait in the living room for a few moments. He left and called the physician who served as the informal chairman of the Guest House board. "Can we have a child here as a resident?" he asked. "I mean, is there anything in our charter that forbids it?"

The doctor said he knew of nothing in their tax-exempt, charitable franchise that would limit residency to adults, but he added that, to qualify, the child would have to have AIDS, since that was what people in the community were told when they were asked for contributions. Warrick Allen said he believed the boy qualified on that count. The doctor said they would need to know for certain. "But, in the meantime," he added, "I suppose we just got ourselves a baby."

Cynthia recalled that when Daphne arrived back at their crude hovel, she seemed more buoyant than her sister had seen her in a long time. Daphne explained what she had done, what had happened to the boy, and why. "You will understand it better when you become a mother," Daphne told Cynthia.

Even Ruth Khumalo expressed her approval of the arrangement, which surprised her daughters. Her sad experiences over the previous weeks, the rigors of her life since she had packed up and left the settlement, had left her increasingly surly. She was seldom pleased, and almost nothing made her happy. Still, that day she told Daphne that she thought she'd done the right thing.

In Houghton that morning, after Daphne departed, Warrick Allen hoisted the boy to his hip and walked into the den, where three or four of the residents were watching television. "Okay, guys," he said, "say hello to your new little brother—and I'm sure you'll all be pleased to know that you've just become charter members of the Guest House Baby-Sitters' Club." The men were mildly enthusiastic. One of them asked the boy's name.

"Nkosi," he answered. He pronounced it tentatively, not sure he had heard it right. He could not remember the other name Daphne had mentioned.

"His name is just Nkosi," he told the dying men.

The boy became an instant star. He was coddled and cuddled and considerably spoiled, not only by Gail and the other volunteers but also by the residents, the men who had come to the Guest House to die. Among them was a former South African Airways pilot, a burly middle-aged man who tried to monopolize the tiny newcomer's presence in their group. The other residents often protested that he kept the child to himself. There were constant arguments over who would feed him, who would change his diapers, who would give him his bath, who would put him to bed, but the pilot was accustomed to the privilege of command, and he usually prevailed. For most of his years, the man had led a tortured existence as a citizen of two separate and distinctly different worlds. In one he was the stereotypically macho bachelor, a stud in aviator glasses who wrestled jumbo jets through sunshine and storm to glamorous destinations. In the other he was a gay man existing precariously on the margins of society. In neither of his worlds had children been a part of his life. To those who witnessed it, his nearly manic affection for the boy seemed a desperate effort to compensate, in the brief time that remained to him, for that absence, to exploit this opportunity to be a father. Early or late, no matter what time of day Gail arrived at the old mansion, the odds were good that the boy and the pilot would be together—stretched out on the floor of the foyer playing with little plastic airplanes, making engine noises in their throats as they lifted them and landed them on the carpet, or watching cartoons on television or simply relaxing on a couch, the tiny black child perched comfortably in the white man's lap.

It was a good memory for Gail, given all the difficulties she and the other sponsors were encountering trying to keep the Guest House afloat. They were only a small cadre, and the financial burden was seriously stretching their resources. With the prevailing cultural antipathy toward homosexuality, fundraising had been problematic from the outset. There were, they found, a finite number of people in Johannesburg who were willing to write checks for the care and feeding of dying gay men. That well had eventually run dry, leaving Gail and the other volunteers to cover the mounting costs themselves.

"There was never a shortage of people willing to donate their time," she later said. "Sure, it was a small and very limited

pool, but everybody in it was quite determined to do every
thing they could."

The money, however, was an entirely different matter. No
one on the board was wealthy, and only a few who had committed themselves to the survival of the place had any surplus
of discretionary funds to contribute to the pot—certainly not
in those days, given the ravaged and deteriorating economy of
the country.

Eventually the time frame they used to measure their financial survival dwindled from months to weeks to days. As
the red ink mounted, Gail and the others discovered, to their
disappointment and dismay—if not their surprise—that they
were just about the last and only people in Johannesburg who
really cared in the least about South African men infected with
AIDS and facing an inevitable death alone. "The overall attitude," Gail later said, "was that all these guys were queers,
queens and fags who had sentenced themselves to death—and
the sooner they were gone, the better."

Alan had been sympathetic and supportive in those hard
times. Like the pilot, Gail had also been drawn to Nkosi and
had often brought him back to her house on Saturdays and
Sundays, simply to provide him with a change of scenery, she
said; Alan hadn't minded in the least. The pilot always objected, of course. "He raised holy hell," she recalled, but the
boy seemed to look forward to his time with Gail and her family, floating in the backyard pool, lazing about with the dog and
the cats, being thoroughly pampered and spoiled by their
daughter and her son, and becoming better acquainted with
Alan, watching cartoons on television from his lap.

"He was such an engaging child, so charming, really quite irresistible," Gail later said, "and of course we all immediately fell in love with him and began to bond with him. And almost before we knew it, we had all begun to accept him as a natural, if only a temporary, weekend part of the family."

In the meantime the future of the Guest House was looking increasingly bleak. Soon the cupboards would be bare, the coffers empty. There simply was not enough money to pay the rent, to pay for the utilities, to buy food and fuel. In mid-January 1992, the board decided there was no alternative but to close the doors. What had begun with such a flood of goodwill and compassion was ending in a flood of debt. "It was agonizing," Gail said. "The pain and sadness of trying to squeeze out one more day, one more hour, yet knowing all along that it could not be done. And the men we had brought there, all those poor, miserable, dying men—they were all seriously traumatized."

In a country and in a culture that had rejected and punished them for what they were, the men of the Guest House had been exhilarated and grateful to have somehow discovered a place that provided unconditional acceptance. They had finally found a few people who would offer them gentle care and companionship and comfort—and suddenly the plug was about to be pulled on all of them.

Gail noticed that the pilot and the boy began spending even more time together as the board and the other volunteers made frantic efforts to find suitable accommodations for the residents. Although the house's population had dwindled over the months—there had been a few deaths—placing the dozen or so who remained was no small task. Yet, one by one, over the days remaining in the skeleton budget, they were all parceled out—to a hospital here, a private home there, until just the boy remained. Under the circumstances, only one solution presented itself.

"He can come with me," Gail told the board.

No one objected.

As the last of the men left the mansion, Warrick Allen packed the boy's belongings and drove him out to Daveyton, explained to his family what had happened to the Guest House, and told them that Gail had offered to take Nkosi into her own family. Daphne agreed. She told Warrick Allen not only that was she still unable to care for him by herself, but also that there were times when she feared for her life because people knew she had AIDS.

It was not a legal adoption, simply an informal arrangement between two women who cared deeply for the boy. "There was never any doubt in my mind," Gail said later, "that Daphne loved him and that however painful it might have been to send him to our house, she only wanted the best for him."

Warrick Allen left Nkosi with his family in the squatters' camp for a few days so that he could celebrate his third birthday there with them.

It was the middle of South Africa's summer, and Gail's PR firm was under contract to a Russian automobile company, promoting the introduction of a new car model in South Africa. On February 8, the day she had planned to drive to Daveyton to pick up the boy, she had also arranged for the automotive writer from one of the local newspapers to test-drive one of the cars. Unfortunately, it ran out of fuel on the road. After urgent calls back and forth between the reporter and Gail's office, she had driven her own car out to find him and bring him a five-gallon can of gasoline. Then she made hasty arrangements with Warrick Allen to retrieve the boy.

Alan was at home that afternoon, comfortably ensconced on the couch in their living room, enjoying the last few pages of a novel, when he was interrupted by a loud knock on the door. "I opened it, and there was this chap standing there holding the boy in one arm and a plastic bag in the other," Alan recalled. "The *chap* was Warrick Allen. And the chap said to me, 'He's all yours,' and just handed him over. Just like that. I had no idea we were expecting him." It was typical Gail, he said, not to have told him that they were taking the boy in on more than a temporary basis. "When she made up her mind to do anything, she did it whether anybody else approved of it or didn't," he said. "It wasn't necessary for her to get an okay from anybody else."

When Gail arrived home later that afternoon, Alan asked why she hadn't informed him of her decision or at least consulted him about it. She said she had intended to discuss it with him but that, with everything going on, it had simply slipped her mind. There was no argument. Alan did not seriously object to the boy's presence in the house and in fact was pleased to have him. But it was just another of the telling moments he would remember after their marriage crumbled.

Yet, though there had been no vote when Gail had decided that the boy would live in their home, on that first evening in February 1992, they had all agreed—Gail and Alan, Nicolette and Brett—that it was as though he had always been there.

With one knock on the door, the four of them had been in-
stantly transformed into a family of five. The tiny Zulu boy
who had never known a real home or a genuine family finally
had both, complete with a mother and father, a big brother
and sister, a dog and several cats, a swimming pool and a
bright, sunlit room of his own. With his new life came a new
name: Xolani Nkosi became Nkosi Johnson.

By whatever name he was called, his prognosis was still
discouragingly dim. The doctors to whom Gail immediately
took the boy were unanimous in their view that there was very
little hope. He was just barely three years old, and they estimated that he had a year or so to live. Everything they knew
about children born with the AIDS virus told them that many
would not live beyond their first birthday, and most would
die within three or four years. They advised Gail that perhaps, with compassionate care and treatment, strict hygiene,
a healthy environment, and a sensible diet, the life expectancy
of such unfortunate children—including Nkosi—might be
slightly extended, but not by much.

"Take good care of him," one of the physicians advised Gail,
"because the odds are you're not going to have him all that long."

FIVE

Xolani Nkosi was three years old that February; Nelson Mandela had been out of prison for two years. It's fair to say that during this time both boy and country were struggling to make the best of an uncertain future in the face of a grim inheritance from the past.

Whenever the marathon negotiations between the old regime and Mandela's African National Congress appeared to stall, a chorus of black voices was raised, impatiently demanding a solution, threatening an escalation of armed insurrection if none was forthcoming. Sporadic episodes of violence were precipitated by unhappy blacks. Meanwhile a hard-line minority of whites, mainly Afrikaners, showed a similar volatility, holding noisy, rabble-rousing rallies that were often bellicose calls to arms for the true believers in apartheid, or at least for those sufficiently fervent to try to defend and preserve it at the point of a gun.

Gail Johnson kept up with it all. It was, of course, un- avoidable for her and every other South African with access to any media outlet, but she couldn't allow herself to be dis- tracted. The clearest summons she recognized that month was in the doctors' bleak prognosis for the boy's survival. Not that she was surprised. Daphne had candidly told Warrick Allen that first morning at the Guest House that Nkosi was infected, that he had *ingculaza*. The doctors' confirmation did nothing to dampen either Gail's optimism or her enthusiasm for in- serting herself into this boy's life. It was almost as if what the doctors told her about the boy's miserable condition, in- cluding the fact that he had tuberculosis, served as a call to combat. It was a war she would wage fiercely for years to come: the day-to-day struggle not only to keep him alive but to enhance his life, to provide him with the essentials for a *good* life.

"This will sound a bit odd, I'm sure," she would recall, "but there were times when I thought I believed I could somehow do what no one else had ever done, which was to change the outcome of his infection." She *thought* she *believed:* an interest- ing if illogical paradigm, constructed as much for her own benefit as for the boy's. She understood that ahead of both of them lay mountains of considerable pain and anguish, yet by persuading herself that there was a worthwhile objective, she *thought* she *believed* she could bear it herself, *thought* she *be- lieved* she could help him endure it as well. "The truth, of course, is that I was never really and truly convinced that in the long run I could save him or cure him," she said. "I only acted as though I could, and that kept me going."

Right from the very beginning, from the first day Nkosi came to live with her, one of the tools she deemed essential for her task was a commodity that was in short supply in the South Africa of those days: laughter.

She remembered having read several magazine and newspaper articles about medical studies that testified to laughter's therapeutic qualities. "I suppose by then everybody had seen this theory or at least heard about it," she later said. "It wasn't rocket science. It was pretty simple, really. It just suggested that laughing—you know, happiness, merriment, enjoying yourself, having a good time as much of the time as possible, however you want to describe it—almost always has a beneficial effect on anyone, whether sick or not." Having very few alternatives beyond the medication available to her—mainly antibiotics but little else—Gail decided on laughter as her basic approach to Nkosi's health and welfare. Even though he was little more than an infant when he was brought to her house to live—a tiny runt of a child, barely walking and not yet talking—she was determined that all his waking hours would be filled with joy, with songs and games and, if necessary, downright silliness. To this task, Gail immediately recruited all the other members of her household—Alan, Brett, and Nikki, too. Once enlisted, each became a participant in her project, including her naturally reserved husband.

"We had no real plan to speak of, and most of the time we had no idea what we were doing," she said. "But we were all damn well willing to try. You wouldn't believe what fools we

made of ourselves in those days: down on our knees on the
floor with him, or cuddled up on the couch, always talking to
him, tickling him—he loved that, the tickling and the touching—lots of Eskimo kisses, always pretending that whatever
Nkosi did or whatever the look Nkosi happened to have on his
face was absolutely hilarious, breathtakingly funny, and we
were always exploding into fits of insane laughter. Sometimes
we faked it, and because it wasn't altogether genuine, we had
to become fairly accomplished actors. Clowns, really. Not
suited to tragedy, of course."

It turned out to be a mighty powerful regimen, not to
mention a wholesome and effective approach to the early nur-
ture and development of any child Nkosi's age. Moreover, it
seemed to work both ways—for them *and* for him. Through
their application of such an informal and lighthearted therapy,
Gail and her family were inevitably bonding with the boy. Simultaneously, as he was becoming accustomed to the sense of
safety, to the warm and reassuring blanket of love and security
they were providing, he was also having the time of his young
life. In a word, he was having *fun*—and that seemed to go a
long way in terms of both his own adjustment to a different
environment and his physical health. It came as no surprise to
Gail or anyone else in the family that eventually Nkosi's first
recognizable words were "Ha, ha, ha," three in a row, which
brought peals of laughter from the rest of the family, of course,
which prompted another ha, ha, ha from him—and so on.

"I think that if anyone had been eavesdropping or spying on
us," Gail said, "they would have had good reason to believe

they had stumbled on a bloody asylum, a houseful of stark, raving maniacs."

From a certain perspective, that conclusion would have been appropriate. Given the brittle state of Gail and Alan's marriage, it was quite insane for them to increase the psychological and emotional pressures on them by embracing as a full-time responsibility a child suffering from an incurable disease. Gail had not sugarcoated for her family the doctors' views when she returned from Nkosi's first major examination. For the couple to involve their children as well simply compounded the craziness and widened the circle of eventual trauma. Yet, over and over, it always seems to be the case that without at least a little "madness," such against-the-odds commitments are rarely made—or kept. Consider, for example, the number of American families who adopt and successfully raise a number of children with special needs, or of ethnic descent other than their own. They have been successful only because common sense was ignored. Life experience and logic were sent to the back of the line. The same was true for the Johnsons: If Gail and her family had not been able to make a leap beyond the limits of rational thinking, they would never have welcomed Nkosi into their home. They well understood from past experience that raising a child anywhere is always tough, and raising a child of any color in the unstable environment of South Africa in those days even more so. For a white family in Johannesburg to take in a Zulu boy infected with AIDS was nothing less than sheer lunacy.

Still, for the Johnsons and for the boy, it was a lunacy

inspired by love. And certainly with their meticulous devotion to every aspect of his needs—from medication to diet, from hygiene to personal habits—his future was at least more promising than the doctors' verdict.

But all the laughter in the world could not eliminate Nkosi's physical problems or the relentless necessity of dealing with them every day. His little pooch of a belly was not the product of malnutrition—he was being regularly provided with a wholesome and well-rounded diet—but rather the result of chronic infections in his liver and spleen. Each of the organs was perhaps twice its normal size. There was also his chronic diarrhea, which compounded the problem of his toilet training. His nose and throat were still heavily congested, as they had been since his early days with Daphne. "It seemed that mucus was his best friend," Gail would recall. He was constantly sniffling and snuffling, his tonsils and adenoids were enlarged, and there were blisters on the inside of his mouth. His breathing was still labored, and a pitiful rasp still emanated from his concave chest. His cough refused to go away, and often at night he would cry out with the pain of earaches. In addition, no matter how much healthy food was put before him, his appetite was as small as his birdlike body. He ate sparingly, and consequently his weight gain was slight.

One afternoon a reporter for a local newspaper came to interview the family for a feature story. The reporter's story described Gail as "the Mother Teresa of Johannesburg" and mentioned not only that she had been one of the principals in the Guest House but that she was also considering trying to open a second care center for women with AIDS and their children. Gail told the journalist she was elated that Nkosi's tuberculosis was in remission, but he had sores on his face and a serious breathing problem. More important, she said, his white-cell count had dropped dramatically. "Maybe we'll reach a crisis point this year," she said.

When she read the story in the paper, she regretted having suggested that things were not going well with Nkosi. "It was true that I always had this feeling of fear and dread about his future," she later said, "but it was stupid of me to express it." From then on, Gail resolved not to be discouraged, or at least not to mention it. "But I have to be honest," she said. "There were quite a few days when I just didn't quite know what to do next, when I really had no idea what was the best way to go. But I also understood every single day that if I didn't do something—maybe it was only to change his diaper or to cuddle him or talk to him or coax him to eat something or take his medicine—nobody else would."

She recorded in a diary the slightest change in his condition. She was faithful to a regimen of bimonthly doctor visits for the boy, ever by his side, comforting him as the nurses extracted yet another vial of blood from his skinny arm, drying his tears, reassuring him as he was poked and prodded on the examination table, as tongue depressors were inserted into his mouth and down his throat. Whatever the cost to her business or to the other members of her family, she was there for him, with him, the sound of her rough-textured, cigarette alto soothingly in his ear, her hand wrapped around his.

By his fourth birthday in 1993, a corner seemed, if not to have been turned, at least to have been approached. There had been something of a payoff. Not much, admittedly, but for Gail and the doctors, even a little was a lot. A few of Nkosi's infections had eased off a bit, including the tuberculosis, and his breathing was steadily improving—though the congestion and diarrhea remained and would never quite be eliminated. Most promising of all, he was eating much better and gaining some weight. "We celebrated every damned ounce," Gail later said.

As miraculous as it may have seemed, during those first couple of years with the Johnsons, this terribly small and gravely ill child became a genuine little boy. He was full of mischief and curiosity, and although his stamina and energy were necessarily limited by his condition, he was usually on the move, full of questions, demanding answers and attention. He was talking by then, calling everyone in his new family by name. Alan was "Daddy," Gail was "Mummy," Brett was "Bwett," Nicolette was "Neeki." Duke, the big shepherd, was "Juke," and the cats . . . well, no one ever did manage to decipher Nkosi's garbled pronunciation of the names of the cats, the only members of the family who weren't won over by his charms—or anyone else's. "They probably thought he was speaking Zulu," Gail said.

Even as the boy's health seemed to be improving, prospects for South Africa's future also seemed to be looking up. Mandela and de Klerk were jointly awarded the Nobel Peace Prize for cobbling together a multiracial interim government that worked fairly well and carried the country into the national

elections of 1994. It was the first time everyone could vote—
including blacks—and although the campaign was marred by
episodes of violence, especially among the Zulus, it was won
handily by Mandela's party, the African National Congress,
which made him the country's new president.

"I had no idea what would happen," Gail recalled, looking
back, "and although I did sort of believe in the myth and, you
know, the magic of Mandela, I managed to maintain a very
practical perspective on the future. You know, I just thought
that almost anything would certainly be better than the way
South Africa had been for so long—but that it would be fool-
ish to hope that the country would be dramatically changed
for the better overnight."

It was the same hopeful approach she had taken with Nkosi.
Any progress in his condition, even the smallest measure, was
better than none and certainly better than the way he had been
when he'd first been delivered to their door.

At first Daphne would call the Johnsons' house every ten
days or so. Then there were a few weekends when Gail drove
Nkosi out to visit his biological family near Daveyton. They all
seemed pleased to have him around, and his sister, Mbali, was
always delighted, but Gail found conditions in the dirt-floor
shack so deplorable, deemed them so detrimental to the boy's
health and hygiene, that she was reluctant to plan any addi-
tional sleepovers. "I would have continued them if Ruth or
Daphne had insisted," she said, "but they didn't, so I didn't."

On those occasions when Daphne dropped in on the Johnsons—no easy task for her, given the spotty transportation and
the considerable distance from Daveyton to Johannesburg—

she often said she was greatly surprised by how much change she was able to observe in Nkosi, by how much brighter and livelier her son seemed to be. On one visit she was so impressed that she asked Gail if perhaps the doctors could have been mistaken in their diagnosis.

Nkosi called his biological mother "Mummy" as well and did not seem at all confused about the identities and roles of the two main women in his life. "That was one of the many things I found really remarkable about him," Gail later said. "It was instinctive, I think. He just accepted the arrangement. She was his mother, yes, but so was I." Eventually, whenever the three of them were together, he distinguished between them by calling her "Mummy Gail" while Daphne was simply "Mummy."

Even though he had been separated from his mother at such an early age, their reunions were poignant. Daphne would hold Nkosi frequently, feed him on the rare occasions he was hungry, help with his medicine, and change his diapers. When she talked with him, she would tell him about the rest of his family, including his aunts and uncles, his grandmother and his sister, of whom he could have little memory. Sometimes mother and child would just sit on the couch together and watch cartoons on television. Often Gail tried to disappear, to leave them alone.

Nearly every time Daphne came to see Nkosi, Gail asked her if she was still satisfied with the arrangement. Daphne always said she was, and she showed no inclination to alter it. Gail also noticed that Daphne's health was deteriorating. Her voice was softer, and her strength was waning.

According to her younger sister, Cynthia, things were becoming increasingly difficult for Daphne in those years. Although she was not steadily employed, she was still working at odd jobs here and there, in Daveyton and even as far away as the suburbs of Johannesburg, but her lack of energy was a major impediment. She would return to the family's shanty totally exhausted, almost unable to undress for bed. Daphne tried to be attentive to her daughter's needs, but her fatigue was often overwhelming. Mbali was going to school in Daveyton by then and doing quite well in her studies, Cynthia said, but Daphne was ill equipped to help with her homework, to see to her clothing, to awaken her and get her breakfast, to see her off each day. "So the rest of us tried to pitch in," Cynthia recalled.

Among the neighbors who were aware of Daphne's condition or at least suspected it, some hostility remained and, from time to time, materialized into threats, both direct and veiled, against her and the other members of her family. In response, Cynthia said, Daphne "was always talking about maybe going back home to Newcastle, so that maybe she could start over again without anyone knowing who she was or at least knowing that she was infected." The anonymity she had discovered and cherished on her first trip to Johannesburg the year before Nkosi was born was still a warm memory for her, a relatively happy time to which she wished she could return.

Most often, however, Daphne simply plodded through each day as though she were climbing one of the great long hills of Zululand, moving more slowly from one day to the next, accepting each one on its own dark terms, absent any real plans or hopes, with no dream of a better future in Egoli, the city of gold.

G ail continued to be as active as possible with the friends with whom she had worked at the Guest House, but she had her hands full trying to look after Nkosi in addition to ful- filling her other commitments. Her household had adjusted to the extra demands of Nkosi's presence, and a sense of normal- ity reigned. With difficulty she carved out a few hours each week to contribute time to several AIDS support groups in Jo- hannesburg. She had rich memories of the Guest House, but its failure still haunted her, and she was never quite able to dis- miss from her mind the need to furnish a safe place for victims of the disease.

As the years passed, her attention began to focus on pro- viding a shelter for mothers who were dying of AIDS and their children. Daphne had recounted for her the unfortunate ex- periences she'd had with her employer, with her doctor, and with her hostile neighbors; these stories, as much as anything else, persuaded Gail that something had to be done for women in such circumstances. She had read accounts of the murder of women who openly declared themselves HIV-positive and had encountered a similar if less extreme prejudice in her own life. Because she had not concealed or disguised Nkosi's condi- tion, many of the other mothers in her circle of friends were reluctant to allow their children to be around him, declining to bring them to pool parties at the Johnsons' house or to his birthday celebrations. "I remember one of them saying to me,

'I just don't think it's a good idea, because my boy's a biter,'"
Gail recalled. "Then she smiled sweetly and said, 'I hope you
understand.'"

Gail understood that the fear of AIDS victims was a fear
based on widespread ignorance of the disease, the same fear
that resulted in the daily punishment and social rejection of its
victims in South Africa, in all its many ethnic communities.
Because she thought Nkosi needed some regular contact with
other children, and given the fact that almost no other mothers would bring their children to play with him or welcome
him into their homes, she decided to enroll him in a neighborhood nursery school and kindergarten. Because she did not
try to hide his condition from those who ran the little school,
she was told in no uncertain terms that Nkosi was not welcome. Gail was repulsed by their attitude. Somehow, someday, she told herself, she would find a way to create a solution,
not only for Nkosi but for at least some of the other women
and children like him and his mother. Gail also decided that
when she did, the first resident would be Daphne.

By the end of 1995, President Nelson Mandela had dis-
missed his wife, Winnie, from a government post to
which he had appointed her. Her public behavior had struck
him and many of his closest advisers as increasingly unacceptable. She had been charged with kidnapping and implicated in
at least one murder. Her statements on politics and the government's policies grew less palatable to the ANC and to
Mandela himself. Within a few months, the two had filed for

divorce. Most of their mutual friends believed that their long marriage had been wounded far beyond repair by the decades of their separation; many thought it was as much a casualty of apartheid as any of the system's other, more obvious victims. Although their public estrangement captivated a great many South Africans—news of it was garishly splashed across the front pages of the country's newspapers on a daily basis—it was seldom raised as a topic of conversation in Gail and Alan Johnson's house. Their own marriage was in serious trouble, and the Mandelas' marital problems struck too close to home.

In 1996 the Mandelas were officially divorced. When Gail read the news, it occurred to her that despite the public airing of their rather badly soiled laundry, they seemed to have handled it with a great deal of dignity. She hoped that when she and Alan were divorced, they might deal with it in the same way. She did not believe that it was a question of if but of when, and she sensed that Alan felt precisely the same way. It seemed only a matter of time.

Meanwhile they focused themselves on other concerns—on his business, on her business, on family business such as teaching Nkosi to read and write and coping with their daughter's adolescent needs, on trying to stay afloat financially in the ongoing South African recession. On everything and anything *but* their crumbling relationship.

Both of Gail's adopted parents had died by then, and she had suddenly taken an intense interest in her own origins. She spent considerable time poring over the records at the hospital where she was born and at the home to which she'd been taken as an infant. She finally learned her biological mother's name and eventually located her in Cape Town, where she was still teaching in the local school system. Gail contacted her, and a meeting was arranged, which, given the circumstances, seemed to go rather splendidly for both of them. Gail found her mother to be a soft-spoken woman, a kind and gentle person who showed great interest in her daughter's life, in the son-in-law she'd never met, the grandchildren she'd never even known she had. She was especially touched by her daughter's story of how she had also become pregnant before marriage, and she expressed regret that, unlike Gail, she herself had chosen to give her child up for adoption. And she was greatly impressed with her daughter's willingness to embrace the young Zulu child.

The five different medications Nkosi was given each day were having some effect, and his condition was stable, if not greatly improved. Still, his weight was a problem, and he was still wearing clothes meant for a two-year-old. There had been only one accident: a time when he fell, bit his lip, and bled a great deal. In the normal course of events, Gail wore no gloves or other protective garb when dealing with him.

Alan enjoyed spending time with Nkosi. He taught him to appreciate football—what Americans call soccer—convincing him that the only team worthy of anyone's loyalty and support was not in South Africa but back in England. "Leeds United is number one," Nkosi would say along with him. Alan also took him often to see motor-sports events at the track in Kyalami, and Nkosi loved them—loved the roar of the cars at full throttle, loved being in the pits to which Alan, with his television producer's credentials, was admitted. When races outside South Africa were televised, the two of them would always watch, sitting together on the couch. Soon the boy had settled on Michael Schumacher, the German driver who was dominating the international Grand Prix competition, as his favorite.

By the end of 1996, the Johnsons' marriage finally reached its end. It was a relatively amicable separation. Alan moved out, Gail kept the house where they had lived for so many years—and both tried to go on with their lives. For their part, Brett and Nicolette seemed relieved that the decision had at last been made.

For Nkosi, however, it was a different matter. He had never known any father except Alan. They had closely bonded during the time they spent together, and not having him around was a difficult adjustment for the boy. "I'm sure for Alan, too," Gail later said.

Brett found more time for Nkosi in his schedule—he was studying engineering by then—and Gail and Alan tried to compensate by arranging frequent visits and continuing the outings to the races and soccer matches. Eventually, Nkosi made his peace with it.

Alan was happily in attendance at Brett's wedding in February 1997, soon after Nkosi's eighth birthday. It was a gala affair, at which Nkosi was dressed to the nines in a miniature tuxedo, complete with a frilly shirt. Serving as the ring bearer, he proudly followed his big brother and his bride down the aisle. Photographs from the wedding show him grinning from ear to ear, a very happy little Zulu boy who was now a genuine member of this Johannesburg family.

B ut by February 1997 it was also true that Daphne's health
was deteriorating alarmingly. Gail was able to calibrate
her steady decline by the increasing difficulty she had in simply
trying to lift her almost weightless little boy. "I remember
thinking each time she came that the next time she wouldn't
be able to pick him up," Gail later said. "I also began to think
that each visit could very well be the last one."

Daphne had surprised everyone by somehow finding the
strength to make the arduous journey back to her birthplace in
Newcastle, whether intending to remain there or simply to re-
visit her origins for a while before returning to the family's
shack in the squatters' camp near Daveyton, it was never clear.
"She didn't really explain it to me," Cynthia said. There, in what
had once been Zululand, in the place where Daphne and both
her children had been born, her condition suddenly worsened.
And it was there, after a few days, that she died. The cause of
death was officially listed as respiratory infection, a common
enough explanation for African victims of AIDS. She went to
her grave without naming the man who had given her and
Nkosi the virus that killed her. She was twenty-five years old.

When Cynthia learned of her older sister's death, she telephoned Gail in Johannesburg and asked whether it would be
better for Nkosi to be informed by Gail or by her. Gail wasn't
certain. She sensed in Cynthia's voice that she preferred to tell
the boy herself, so Nkosi was called to the phone. Several
years later he would tell me his recollections of that moment.

"My auntie said my mummy had gone on a trip to Newcastle," he said, tears welling in his eyes. "Then my auntie said my

mummy had become very sick in Newcastle while she was there."

You already knew she was very sick, didn't you? I asked.

"Yes," said Nkosi. "I already knew my mummy was very sick, and I already knew that my mummy and I both had the same sickness, and I knew we both would die with the same sickness, but I didn't know she would die so soon, and it made me very sad, and I cried a lot when my auntie told me she had gone to heaven and that I would not see my mummy anymore."

Gail would recall that, though his relationship with Daphne had been only episodic, the boy was genuinely heartbroken. Gail consoled him as best she could and asked if he wanted to attend his mother's funeral. "He said yes, he did want to be there," Gail said, "but, to be honest, I don't think he had the slightest concept of what a funeral was, much less death, even less the death of his mother." Two days later she made the long drive to Newcastle with him and delivered him to his grandmother, Ruth, and to Cynthia and his other aunts and uncles, then waited in the car some distance away from the little cemetery where Daphne was to be buried. Years later Nkosi would remember that day in Newcastle quite vividly. He had been only eight years old, yet he would have good reason to remember it for the rest of his own life. He recalled that it was during the service for his mother that his grandmother had pointed out a man he had never seen before, identified him as his father and Mbali's as well, and taken Nkosi by the hand to meet him.

"But he didn't say anything to me," Nkosi said. "He didn't

say he was my father, and he didn't say why he had never come to see me or anything like that, and he didn't touch me or hug me or anything. He just looked at me. I know he was very sad about my mummy's going to heaven. I saw him crying—but he didn't say anything to me. I didn't understand why he wouldn't talk to me, and I didn't understand why he didn't hug me or anything like that, and I don't think he was my father."

O n that sad afternoon, with his mother dead and buried and with no identifiable father present in his life, Nkosi involuntarily joined another family: the enormous family of African children orphaned by AIDS.

On the day Daphne died, there were at least 100,000 AIDS orphans in South Africa alone. In Zambia there were 400,000, or 10 percent of the total population, and in Uganda, more than a million. The approximate number of AIDS orphans on the entire continent at that point was 10 million. It is a staggering number, but considering that more adults are now living with AIDS than have already died from it, over the next few years, probably by 2010, the total is expected to reach 25 million— at least.

Despite his infection, Nkosi might rightly be seen as relatively fortunate, one of the rare kids lucky enough to find a haven and a home. The reality is that the vast majority of African youngsters who lose one or both their parents to the disease are left alone to fend for themselves, to grow up by themselves, to raise younger siblings by themselves, to sacrifice even a limited education for work—if indeed work can be found—and eventually to be buried deeper and deeper in abject poverty, Africa's other killer.

In most of the countries, very little attention is paid to these children, either by the government or by the churches or charities. In a very few places, there are informal arrangements for community care. The AIDS orphans are unofficially adopted by the villages where their parents had lived, by their uncles and aunts and grandparents, or perhaps by close friends or anyone else willing to lend a hand in their care.

In Malawi, for example, the crushing impact of AIDS has added another burden to a country laboring under more than its share. A terrible dry season is followed by a terrible flood season, when rains sufficiently torrential to drown children and small animals wash away village huts, leaving already hungry families homeless as well. Even before AIDS hit, the infant mortality rate in Malawi was desperately high. For the most part, Malawians believe in a benevolent, beneficent deity, but they also believe in other forces, malevolent and evil: witches who can transform themselves into hyenas, or residents of other communities who can destroy their enemies by harnessing floods. Imagine the impact on such a place of an invisible virus that infects and spreads exponentially, that leaves more than 300,000 children without their parents.

In the Malawian village of Mponela, where the community-care approach is the only resource available to the orphans of AIDS, the statistics are overwhelming. In 1997, as the number of weekly funerals mounted, what began as a project involving 50 orphans quickly mushroomed into one with more

than 150—and with no money from the government, not
much prospect for enhancing their lives. All the government
provides there—probably all it *can* provide, given its strapped
fiscal condition—is moral support, a bare-bones policy of encouraging villages to keep the children close to their roots.

It is hardly enough. The wife of the local chief—Grandma
Kaomba, she is called—is the matriarchal head of a family so
devastated and depleted by AIDS that she is single-handedly
caring for at least a dozen orphans, the sons and daughters of
her own dead children and those of other relatives as well. It is
nearly beyond her abilities and her strengths, yet there is no
other way. She is a strong advocate of the community-care approach. She says, "If you take these children away from us and
put them in a home and they grow up with children from different places, different areas, they will lose their culture. They
will not know their roots."

Other, more institutional efforts are being made to deal
with the enormous problem. Although they are few and far
between and cannot hope to cope with the escalating numbers
of orphaned children, they do exist. In another rural setting in
Malawi, for example, an orphanage sponsored by a church
group in California headed by a kindly pair of gentle and dedicated Malawians provides a haven for about thirty children
caught in the same web that trapped and killed their parents,
the same web that has created millions of other orphans like
them. Among the occupants of the home on the day I visited
was a boy named Innocent, the oldest of the group. A bright
and handsome kid, just barely twelve, he was quite aware of
his good fortune in having found a place where, through the

kindness of strangers, he and the others were being fed and clothed, housed and taught.

"My mother was the first to die," he said in soft, liltingly accented English. "And then my father—and now this is all the family I have. I love them, and they love me." It may be an artificial family, with limited means and facilities, but for Innocent and for his new brothers and sisters, it is better than no family at all.

Sooner or later every country in Africa will have to face how it will deal with such children, whether through community-based care or in institutional settings or, most typically at the moment and probably for some time to come, through sheer neglect. But whatever the decision, without some remarkable transformation, none will be able to cope with the numbers. Inevitably, an overwhelming tide of needy children will swamp every country's thinly stretched resources, and as the number of adults who die from AIDS increases exponentially, there will be many fewer African adults to care for Africa's orphans.

In the weeks following Daphne's death, Nkosi sank into a funk, at least a mild depression if not something more serious. He was clearly much grumpier than usual, but he was reluctant to talk to Gail about whatever it was that was bothering him. She was patient, did not press him, and eventually he told her what was on his mind.

Like almost everyone else confronted by a death in the family, the boy had been reminded of his own mortality. For most eight-year-olds, in fact for most everyone, it would have been only a passing shiver, an acknowledgment that yes, there is inevitably an end to life, including one's own. For Nkosi, however, it was different. His grief for his mother was mixed with the recognition that, as he would explain to me years later, his mother's death from AIDS had given him a stark premonition of his own future. As he eventually told Gail, he was not only sad for Daphne but feeling sorry for himself.

"He said he did not want to die," Gail recalled. "I said, 'Nobody does, sweetie, but we all do.'"

It was then that his tears began to flow.

"He said, 'I know that, Mummy Gail. I know that—but I still don't want to die. I want to live to be old, like you.'"

Gail stifled a giggle at this last remark; she was, after all, only forty-eight. She told the boy in the most serious of tones that she and everyone else who loved him would do everything possible to give him a long and happy life. "That seemed to satisfy him," Gail later said, "and before long he was back to being his old self."

He was not a perfect child. He was lackadaisical about his chores—feeding the cats or the dog, cleaning up his room. He complained whenever he had to take his daily medicines. He was as mischievous as any other boy his age, always devising pranks and practical jokes on Gail or Nikki or the maid. In short, despite his origins, despite what had happened to him in the brief span of his life, despite his terminal condition, he was really not an unusual kid.

"He loved jokes, telling jokes," Gail later said, "but he could never remember the punch lines. So he'd start out with this elaborate setup—you know, a dog walks into a bar or something like that—then captivate everybody with the most complicated plot, and always, in the end, he could never remember how the joke ended, which was just as funny, of course, as if he did."

He and Gail had a mutual passion for baths. He loved taking them in extremely hot water, which somehow soothed him. Quite often he joined Gail in her giant whirlpool tub. "Sometimes," Gail said, "he would start running the water before I got home so that it was ready for me and, of course, for him. I never saw a kid so at peace in a bath. He didn't splash around. No horseplay. He just liked to lie back and relax and enjoy it."

It was not all so easy for Gail. The constant attention to Nkosi—to his temperature, to the condition of his bowels, to his blood tests, to his twice-a-month visits to the doctors who were his principal lifelines—was draining for her. And then, one day in 1997—before his mother's death and Brett's marriage—the undersize boy who could be so endearing and exasperating, like all boys, suddenly announced to her that he was tired of spending his days alone with the maid while Gail was out running her business.

"I want to go to school," he told her, "just like everybody else."

Gail was surprised. "Actually, I was stunned. It was the last thing I expected from him—and that's because I stupidly believed we were providing everything any child could want. In fact, what he really wanted, we were not giving him, which was the opportunity to be a child among children."

Her first thought when she heard his request was of his blunt rejection by the nursery school when she had tried to enroll him as a much younger child. Her second thought, in her own words, was, "By God, if that's what he wants, then that's what he gets—even if it kills me."

She kissed him on both his hollow cheeks and told him, "Of course, sweetie. If you want to go to school, you will go to school."

It would not be that simple. Almost nothing in South Africa was simple, not in those days and not now. Nevertheless, his decision and hers would launch them both on a radical course that would change the direction not only of their lives but of their country's as well. Together the two of them— Gail and Nkosi—were about to make a bit of South African history.

SIX

Of all the factors that shaped the course of Nkosi Johnson's life, few would be more important than the innocuous blank lines that followed one of the questions on a standard South African public-school enrollment form. It was included in a section dealing with the applicant's personal-health history, and it asked for information concerning any continuing infectious illnesses, contagious diseases or conditions.

Gail had always been open about Nkosi's infection—with all her friends and neighbors, with the members of her family, and her business associates as well—and with the same honesty, without a moment's hesitation, sitting at her dining-room table that afternoon in February 1997, she filled in the empty lines truthfully, thereby making certain that the authorities at Melpark Primary School were aware of the fact that the little boy applying for enrollment there was HIV-positive.

Looking back at that moment, she said she was absolutely unaware of any impending controversy.

"I wasn't thinking in those terms at all," she said. "Nkosi said he wanted to go to school. Therefore, that's exactly what I wanted, too. The forms were simply a step in that process— but I wasn't going to lie about his condition or conceal it. Why should I do that?"

She hand-carried the papers to the principal's office, returned home, and waited.

By 1997, AIDS was no longer flying under anyone's radar, no longer regarded as some exotic killer stalking and targeting mainly homosexual men. Around the world at least 36 million people were infected, a staggering total in itself. But more astoundingly, in the countries of sub-Saharan Africa, with a population of 270 million, more than 26 million were HIV-positive, nearly 10 percent—and nearly 70 percent of the entire total for the earth. Every day almost 10,000 *new* infections were occurring, and every day nearly 7,000 Africans were dying of the disease—35,000 each week, about 2 million a year. Most of its victims were breadwinners—women and men—each with an average of ten dependents. By 1997, 70,000 African babies were being born HIV-positive every year.

Everywhere I traveled on the continent in those days, in nation after nation, place after place, reporting on this war and that revolution, covering famines and floods and genocidal slaughter, the statistics related to AIDS were as shocking as the body counts from the armed conflicts or natural disasters. Among the most alarming yet sobering numbers I came across was this one: During the 1990s in Botswana, the average life expectancy of residents had been savagely reduced by the virus in less than a single decade from just over 68 years to just under 50 years—and it was still headed downward. Moreover, a third of the adult population of Botswana was infected, and there were already 80,000 AIDS orphans.

I recall a particular afternoon spent in a small village not far from Gaborone, the capital, where the busiest fellow in town—and also the most successful—was a middle-aged man who had once been the local carpenter, paid for a few journeyman jobs of simple construction and repairs. In the previous two years, he had astutely adapted his skills to the building of coffins. He was capable of providing a grieving family with anything from a rough-hewn and inexpensive wooden crate to a range of more ornate, satin-lined caskets, including his top-of-the-line model, which came complete with brass handles and custom-carved figures or religious messages on its polished exterior. Few residents of the village could afford such luxury, and his most popular product was the simplest one, which came in an adult size, about six feet by two, and a much smaller one for the children who were dying. In only the week previous to my visit, he said, in his community of no more than five hundred people, there had been fourteen funerals.

"So, you see, I sell fourteen coffins," he said. In the coming few days, he said, eight more were scheduled, all for local victims of AIDS. Some of the families had already ordered or picked up their coffins. "I am very busy always, day and night," the carpenter said on that humid afternoon outside his little shop. "The disease is very bad, of course. I am not glad for the disease, but for my business now, it is very growing."

All across the continent, similar businesses were thriving, and in South Africa, as in all its neighboring countries, almost everyone in the black community, both in the rural villages and in the townships, knew someone who had died of AIDS or was at least in the long and painful process of doing so. At least 10 percent of South Africa's adult population was fatally infected—half of them still young people, not yet out of their twenties—and one in every five pregnant women was HIV-positive, likely to pass along the virus to her child, as Daphne had infected Nkosi. The nation was quite literally under siege, yet most of its 43 million citizens were still unaware or in denial of the more significant details of the virus: what it was, what it did to the people it infected, how it was transferred from one person to another, how rapidly it was spreading, how it could be prevented. The fledgling government, headed by the African National Congress—Vice President Thabo Mbeki had just become the party's new leader—was saying very little and doing absolutely nothing, behaving as though no public-health crisis, no such threat to its people, existed. Sometime later, after Nelson Mandela had left the presidency and Mbeki had succeeded him, Mandela would express considerable regret about his lack of action in those days and would apologize for not guiding his government into emergency measures. He would also offer this rather amazing explanation of why he had not: because AIDS was primarily a sexually transmitted disease, he was embarrassed to speak of it in public. His service to South Africa was inestimable, yet whatever else he may have done for his country—and his

achievements were many—his inattention to the growing
AIDS crisis was Mandela's most tragic failure.

Gail Johnson felt no such embarrassment. She had just
candidly revealed to the administration of Melpark Primary
School that the little boy applying for admission there was one
of the millions of South Africans who were infected with the
deadly virus.

On the one hand, there was neither a law nor a regulation
that prohibited HIV-positive children from entering South
Africa's public schools. The question had simply never arisen
before. To Gail's delight, at last she heard from the Melpark
principal: Nkosi would be most welcome there. On the other
hand, the parents of the school's students had never been confronted with the possibility that their own kids would be sitting side by side with an infected and probably infectious child,
might be romping together with him on the playground at recess, could be eating lunch with him in the cafeteria, would
inevitably be in close physical proximity to him, perhaps
even . . . touching him. They panicked. Many were fiercely and
adamantly opposed. It was clearly never a question of Nkosi's
race. Melpark was thoroughly integrated and had been for
several years by then. It was simply a matter of fear—of the
ignorance that would pose nearly as great a threat to the country as the virus itself had.

The news of Nkosi's application quickly found its way into
the local media, both broadcast and print—Gail swore she had
nothing to do with it—which soon prompted dozens of parents, black and white, to gather outside the school to protest

his enrollment. One woman carried a hand-printed sign that read, WE DON'T WANT YOU, NKOSI! To allow him into the classroom would be dangerous for their children, they argued, perhaps even fatal. It was unfair, they insisted, to expose their children to a boy who was HIV-positive. And they didn't even realize, Gail later recalled, that he had full-blown AIDS. "He was already pretty far along with it," she said. "It was the real thing, and it was working on his body—and had been for some time."

In fact, the eight-year-old Nkosi had lived longer than any child ever born HIV-positive in South Africa or, as far as anyone knew, anywhere else on the continent. Most died within the first three years. Only a few lived past their fourth birthday and almost none past their fifth. His doctors could not fully explain his remarkable longevity, but they suggested then and later that it was at least partially the product of the loving care and attention he was receiving from Gail and her family, as well as the hygiene of his new home, his healthy diet, and the brace of medications he was taking each day. Not least, they attributed his survival to his stout heart: his emotional and psychological stamina and his steadfast determination to survive.

None of the Melpark parents who opposed his presence in the classroom had any notion of the boy's special gift for the combat to which he had committed himself. They could not be blamed for that, of course. Few South Africans were well versed in the current data about the disease. Just as important, none of them had any idea how formidable Gail Johnson could be once she set her mind to a goal. They were about to find out. When she saw the opposition to Nkosi's admission, she got riled. Her back was up. Daphne's boy—*her* boy, too— would, by God, go to school.

As the controversy heated up, it was accompanied nearly every day by headlines and stories in the Johannesburg papers, on local radio and television, which Gail did nothing to discourage. She was always willing, if not always eager, to sit for as many interviews as were requested of her. She believed she had been drawn into a battle, and for her the interviews were tactical maneuvers. A few mentions of the contretemps began to appear in the national press and in outlets as far away as Cape Town and Durban, even in Gail's old hometown of Pietermaritzburg. Gradually, inexorably, without realizing it or planning it or wanting it, Gail and Nkosi were becoming famous in South Africa.

The Melpark principal, beset by angry letters and telephone calls, was soon wavering in her initial decision to admit Nkosi. At first Gail had been drawn to her, had thought she was trying to do the right thing, to make the best of a very difficult situation. The principal had organized public discussion sessions during which it became clear that the school's faculty and staff were as divided on the question of Nkosi's admission as the protesting parents. Such meetings also demonstrated that several of the parents were not entirely unsympathetic to Nkosi and were looking for ways to make everyone happy. One mother suggested that perhaps the best solution would be to clothe him in a transparent but protective plastic sheath.

"Oh, that was such an elegant idea. Just splendid," Gail re-called sarcastically. "I told her and the rest of them that maybe when we got him all wrapped up, we could change his name. We could call him 'Little Condom.'"

Eventually the harried principal announced that she was scheduling one final meeting of the Melpark parents. Since their children were the ones involved, she said, the parents would be given the ultimate responsibility of guiding the school on its final decision. They could say yes or no to Nkosi, and their opinion would be taken into account. On that evening at the school, after long and impassioned oratory from both sides, replete with fist-shaking and finger-pointing, the vote was taken at last.

Incredibly enough, it was an even split. A tie.

More headlines ensued.

ADMIT AIDS BOY! one Johannesburg tabloid's front page de-manded.

New editorials appeared in the local papers almost daily, most of them favoring Nkosi's admission, asking the city gov-ernment to step in or, in lieu of that, urging the national gov-ernment to act. Local politicians and educators, black and white, took positions, recommending a variety of compro-mises. Letters to the editor poured in.

Gail was on television regularly, defending Nkosi's admis-sion— and he was on television, too. "All I want is to go to school," he said again and again in his soft soprano. "All the other children go to school, and I want to be just like all the other children. I don't want to be alone."

Parents who opposed his admission were regularly on television as well. "I'm sure he's a sweet little boy," one mother said smilingly into the camera. "But I beg of you, don't think only of him. Listen, everybody!" She was no longer smiling. "For God's sake," she shrieked, "think of the other children!"

The principal was *not* on television. Instead she was on the phone with parents and bureaucrats, day after day, call after call.

Finally, acknowledging the enormous pressure for someone in authority to deal with the situation, the national government stepped in. In late February, just in time for the new semester, the South African Parliament, in session in Cape Town, enacted an antibias statute that made it illegal to keep HIV-positive children like Nkosi out of public schools. The parliamentary vote was nearly unanimous, a rare event in that fractious legislature's brief history. Subsequently the South African Department of Education drafted regulations on the nondiscriminatory status and treatment of HIV-positive children in the public schools.

The headlines were jubilant:

AIDS BOY GOING TO SCHOOL!
BRAVE KID CHANGED CONSTITUTION!

At the Johnson residence in suburban Melville, there was a subdued celebration. "When I told him he would finally get his wish," Gail recalled, "that he would go to school just like all the other kids, I expected that there would be a big round of high fives between us. That was his usual style of celebration.

But he didn't say anything. Nothing at all. He just stood there for a moment or two. I suppose he was trying to grasp the significance of what I had just told him—and then all of a sudden his face just exploded into *that* grin. It was the biggest, brightest one I think I ever saw on him. He was one seriously happy little boy."

Because South Africa lies at the bottom of the continent, nearly two thousand miles below the equator, its seasons are the reverse of those in the Northern Hemisphere. Summers in New York and London and Paris are winters in Cape Town and Johannesburg and Durban. When American children run screaming from their schools in June, eager for the freedom of their traditional three-month vacation, South African students are well into their winter term, already having taken their summer holiday from mid-December through mid-March.

Mid-March was only a few weeks away, and Gail and Nkosi hurried to prepare for what he anticipated would be the biggest moment of his life: his first day in school. He had already taken tests that showed him to be capable of studying at the third-grade level. Nevertheless, in the interim between the decision by the Parliament and the beginning of the new term, he and Gail—and, from time to time, Nikki—spent hours at home honing his reading, writing, and mathematics skills. He was certainly bright enough and quite eager; the single most significant impediment to normal learning was his fatigue. He tired easily, and when he was tired, his concentration flagged. When his focus failed him, he much preferred to sit on the couch with Nikki and watch soap operas, like *Days of Our Lives* and *The Young and the Restless.*

When at last the big morning came, Gail helped him get dressed in his new white shirt, dark tie, and blue blazer with the Melpark crest on the breast pocket—all the kids wore uniforms in South African schools—and walked with him to the corner across from Melpark Primary. The sidewalks were jammed with other parents and noisy children. Cars and vans crowded the curbs, dropping off kids.

Gail remembered the moment quite well. "When we stopped there, he looked up at me and, with that smile of his, he said to me, 'You can go home now, Mummy. I'll be just fine.'"

She let go of this hand, left him there, turned away, and headed home. But she could not resist stealing a quick glance over her shoulder to watch him heading across the street, into the jumbled mass of students. "Even though there were a few tears in my eyes, I could see that for sure it looked like he really belonged there."

And with very few glitches, it turned out that, just as Nkosi had assured her he would be, he *was* fine.

Later he gave me his slightly sanitized version of how that sunny Monday came about. "I didn't start to school until the second term because they didn't know what to do with me," he said. "They were worried that if I was to fall and start bleeding, the children would be frightened of me and would run away from me instead of coming up to me and saying, 'Nkosi, can I help you?'

"They had doctors come to the school and talk to the teachers, and they also taught some of the children's mothers about the responsibility of AIDS. Then the teachers and everybody thought about it and decided that yes, it was fine for me to go to school, and so they let me go, which made me very happy and made Mummy Gail happy, too.

"The first day of school, the newspapers took pictures of me in my new uniform. It was a nice day, but I was a little scared because I had no friends at all. I didn't tell anyone that I have AIDS, but I think they knew. There was one boy who I'm sure didn't like me. That first day he greeted me, but if I went near him, he moved away. If I touched other boys, he said, 'Don't go near him. He's got that sickness.' But one of the boys— he's my friend; his name is Aubrey—he said to him, 'Why not?' He told that boy that I am not dangerous.

"I made lots of other friends, too, and most of them also understood."

By the time we had this particular conversation, a few years later, Nkosi had grown quite sanguine about his experience in the classroom, had come to treat it as something fairly routine, always complaining, for instance, about the amount of homework he was assigned every night. Still, he seemed well aware of what his admission to Melpark had meant on a broader scale.

"The schools, I think they know more about AIDS now, but Mummy Gail says that if it wasn't for me, kids with AIDS wouldn't even be allowed in. That would have been terrible, I think, because children with HIV also need to learn and to look after themselves."

In addition to Aubrey, one of the friends Nkosi quickly made was a white classmate named Eric Nichols, a stocky, solidly built boy who more or less took the tiny Nkosi in hand and became both his companion and his champion. Of his own volition, Eric chose to share a desk with Nkosi, and if other students complained about Nkosi's presence, probably reflecting their parents' views, Eric patiently explained to them that they were not at risk. He presented them with obvious object lessons, touching Nkosi's face with his hands, even placing an arm around his narrow shoulders. If others teased Nkosi about his size, Eric took them to task and asked them to try to understand that Nkosi could not help being small, that, like the rest of them, he had nothing to do with how tall or short he was, that his stunted size was simply a result of his condition. If Nkosi was having a problem with his studies, Eric was helpfully at his side in study periods, serving as his at-school tutor, and on many afternoons he came to Nkosi's house to assist him with homework.

"Eric is my very best friend in the whole world," Nkosi would say.

Over so many generations of South Africa's troubled history, the country has produced an abundance of heroes, from Nelson Mandela to Anglican archbishop Desmond Tutu to the Dutch Reformed clergyman Beyers Naude. Eric Nichols deserves to be counted among them.

In the next three years at Melpark Primary, Nkosi would have but one accident. During recess one afternoon, as he was running on the playground, he fell and cut a gash inside his mouth. The bleeding was handled with care but also with ca-

sual aplomb by his teachers and the staff. Moreover, his aca
demic performance in the classroom was promising, his grades
quite satisfactory.

In mid-June, on his first report card, his teacher wrote this:

He is "self-assured and content, usually polite and friendly,
quiet and calm. He carries out instructions, concentrates
well, works at a good pace and is eager to listen. He is able to
make good observations, he can implement activities well and
likes to participate. He always tries hard and communicates
well. His functional work is correct. He has good word recognition and works reasonably with numbers. He always tries his
best."

Her conclusion was that "Nkosi Johnson has worked very
hard this term, with pleasing results."

Then, as a postscript, Mrs. Hastings added a congratula-
tory note to the newest, smallest, and most famous student in
her class: "Well done, Nkosi."

Gail was pleased but not surprised, for she recognized in
the teacher's report what she had long known about the boy.
"It was just the way he was. I take no credit for it at all. He always tried hard, no matter what he was doing, and I cannot remember a single instance in which he did not always do his
absolute best. Except when he was supposed to feed the cats,
of course."

At the end of the struggle over Nkosi's admission to the
school, after the Parliament had ruled in his favor and
the Department of Education had issued its guidelines, after

the other parents had ended their protests and resigned them
selves to his presence at Melpark, after Nkosi seemed to have
settled into his third-grade classroom, Gail at last breathed a
long sigh of relief. The weeks of tension had worn her out. She
was smoking far too much, upwards of two packs every day,
and neglecting her diet. She had lost considerable weight, and
she was edgier than usual, much less patient with her friends,
her colleagues, and her family. She was snapping at people
who did not deserve her hostility. "It's a good thing Alan was
gone by then," she later said. "We might have killed each other."

In short, she was a wreck, and she was looking forward to
some peace and quiet, a little time to spend curled up in a
chaise longue near the pool, reading her mystery novels. She
was immensely pleased that, at last, it was all over.

In fact, it had just begun.

I f fame was the price she and the boy had to pay for their
public crusade, its reward was access and opportunity—
and, perhaps more important, credibility. Nkosi's progress in
the classroom was tracked almost daily by the media—the
most frequent adjectives applied to him in the many stories
published in those days were "brave" and "courageous" and, of
course, "cute." For Gail the rather constant coverage allowed
her to begin talking about her favorite subject: the plight of
women like Daphne and children like Nkosi in South Africa.
Because she was so frequently portrayed in the media as a
woman who was valiantly engaged in trying to make some difference for them, someone who had been spunky enough to

take in the HIV-positive son of a woman dying of AIDS, people were beginning to listen to her. She often received invitations to appear and speak at local civic clubs and organizations. She joined the board of a newly formed AIDS-assistance group called MUSE. In a brief span of time, she had become a genuine public person, a familiar face if not yet a household name. Moreover, she was a *popular* public person—and since she had always been completely open with the press about everything in her life, including her illegitimate son and her failed marriage, she had nothing to hide and was therefore immune to sensationalistic tabloid exposés. She was, she thought, scandal-proof. She soon recognized all this new attention for what it was: a perfect opportunity to advance her pet project, the shelter for women and children with AIDS that had been on her mind for years, ever since the closing of the Guest House.

With newfound confidence and energy, she began raising funds, soliciting contributions from individuals and businesses large and small, from churches and civic clubs, from reporters who came to interview her. Her appeal to every potential contributor was simple. She had memorized her presentation, almost always using exactly the same language.

She would begin by quoting from Mandela's eloquent inaugural address, in which he pledged that "never and never and never again shall it be that this beautiful land will experience the oppression of one by the other."

Then, in unvarying language, Gail would make her pitch. I listened to it two or three times and was always impressed.

"Nevertheless, despite President Mandela's vision for our future, there are thousands of South Africans who are being

oppressed," she would say. "All South Africans should understand that black women between fifteen and forty are especially vulnerable in our country, vulnerable not only to HIV
infection but also to the bias and prejudice and isolation it almost always brings. They're often abandoned or already wid-
owed, and the impact on them is absolutely devastating. They
find themselves destitute, ostracized by their communities,
without friends or families and unable to look after themselves and their children. Sometimes, they're the victims of
beatings, and some of them have been murdered. I want you
to know one more thing about them: They need your help."

A little here, a little there—but never a great deal from
anyone or anywhere—and gradually, after a year or so, she
had accumulated sufficient funds to begin to do more than
hope. Her reach was at least approaching her grasp. Alan generously stepped back into the picture by agreeing to organize
and sponsor a charity golf tournament that produced a bit of
money, a small sum, but greatly appreciated.

She put together a board of directors and incorporated the
still-nonexistent shelter as a charitable institution, eligible for
tax-exempt gifts and donations. She recruited friends and associates who had worked with her at the Guest House and,
with her persuasive enthusiasm, enlisted others who'd never
before been active. For all practical purposes, she had shut
down her company by then, and after more than a year of hard
work, and with plenty of help from her colleagues, she finally
found a house large enough for several women and their children but not so fancy as to cost a fortune in rent. It was at

23 Mitchell Street in Berea, a working-class neighborhood of Johannesburg. The deal was done, the lease was signed, the checks were written. All that remained was a name.

"I decided, rather cynically, I suppose, to exploit my boy, to capitalize on all the ink and airtime he was receiving," Gail frankly admitted later. "And, of course, I wanted to honor Daphne in some way as well, since she had really been the chief inspiration for it all. In the end it was a no-brainer. I decided to call it Nkosi's Haven—and everybody seemed to think it was perfect, just about the only name it could possibly have."

Even before it officially opened, and without much effort from Gail, the shelter gathered a full quotient of positive publicity. In the first week of April 1999, President Mandela invited Gail and Nkosi to his official residence in Houghton, not far from the old Guest House to which the desperate Daphne had brought the boy. Like thousands of others in the country, Mandela had heard about Nkosi's Haven. He wrote a small check, gave it to Gail, and presented both of them with a copy of his autobiography, *Long Walk to Freedom*. He had inscribed it, *Best wishes to a lady who cares and to a very brave young man.*

Later Mandela said that during their conversation at the mansion, he had asked Nkosi if he knew what he'd like to be when he grew up. "The boy thought it over for a minute and then said he was not really sure," Mandela recalled, "so I asked him if perhaps he wanted to have my job, to be the president of South Africa. He had a quick answer for that. He said, 'No thank you, sir.' He said he thought that would be much too much work."

At last, with great fanfare, with eight ailing but very happy mothers and five screaming children waiting to move in, with several camera crews and reporters and photographers on hand to record the event, Nkosi's Haven officially opened its doors on April 14, 1999. An exhausted Gail declared, "I feel like I've just given birth."

Nkosi had been excited during the planning and preparation for the shelter, and when it actually opened, he could not have been more blissfully happy. Besides the whirlpool bath in Gail's bedroom, the house that bore his name would soon become his favorite place to be—and the mothers and their children who had sought and found shelter there would immediately become another family to add to his growing list.

Gail remembered the boy's boundless affection for the house in Berea and the people who lived there. "Outside of school, it was the only other place where he could be with people whose skin was the same color and whose condition matched his. All of the mothers were black then, and all of them and a few of the kids either had AIDS or were HIV-positive, and I think Nkosi felt a great kinship with them, if not because of race then certainly because of the commonality of their disease."

On weekdays after school and on Saturdays and Sundays, he was forever clamoring to go to the shelter. "He was like a wannabe rock star with his first album. Proud and vain and eager for everybody to know that this was a place named for him—not for me, not for Mandela, not for Tutu, not for anybody except him—and however badly he'd been spoiled by me and Alan and Nikki and Brett or by any of the rest of the people who had become his family, everybody at the shelter spoiled him that much more."

He had other friends, of course, adults and children, but Gail believed that in his mind, none of them came close to providing the unconditional love and sheer adoration he received when he was present at Nkosi's Haven. "And believe me," Gail said, "he absolutely lapped it up. It was like a drug for him. He soon became addicted."

Out of nowhere Nkosi had suddenly acquired a family that included several younger brothers and sisters, children even smaller than he was, and he was delighted to play the role of the older, taller sibling for a change. Whenever he was there, he happily pitched in with chores, setting the table for meals, helping to feed some of the babies, changing a diaper here and there, cleaning up after dinner or lunch, even occasionally assisting in the dishwashing. In the den—a crowded mishmash of infants' chairs, old couches, and dozens of toys—he proudly read stories to the younger ones or tried to interest them in the jokes he so mangled or introduced them to the questionable joys of his favorite soap operas.

The mothers in residence babied him, indulged him, were completely devoted to him, and so were the helpers Gail had hired to supervise the shelter. When he was there, she said—and he was often there—he was nothing less than "a little prince."

He and Gail had also become nothing less than icons in the international AIDS community. In 1999 they were invited by several groups to come to the United States. The trip excited Gail, but the prospect of traveling that distance with Nkosi was also daunting for her. She knew that even in the best of circumstances, it would be neither simple nor easy. As she was always reminding others, she once again reminded herself that Nkosi was a very sick little boy—and she reminded him of that fact as well, and warned him that being confined for that many hours on an airplane would be difficult for him, especially with his diarrhea. Eased by his daily medication, it had by then become much less severe than when he first came to live with the Johnsons, but it remained an uncomfortable and, for him, an embarrassing part of his life.

"But he wanted so desperately to make the trip," Gail later said. "He wouldn't listen to any of my warnings. It was the first thing on his mind every morning and the last every night. He was totally relentless on the subject. He never stopped. 'Are we going, Mummy? When are we going? Mummy, we have to go. We must go. We absolutely have to go.'"

Eventually Gail agreed. When she applied for his passport, she discovered that his birth had not been registered. As far as the South African government knew, there was no Xolani Nkosi. Gail and the boy were by then known well enough in the country that the normal red tape and the obstacle of his official anonymity were quickly eliminated by kindly bureaucrats at the Foreign Ministry. Although she had never legally adopted him, a passport was issued in the name of Nkosi *Johnson*. He carried it constantly in the days before their departure, took it with him to Nkosi's Haven and showed it around to the mothers and other children, none of whom had any idea what it was or why he was so proud to have it. Worried that he might lose it, Gail tried to confiscate it. He loudly protested, argued with her that it was his private property, promised he'd take good care of it.

"If you want to go to America," she told him, "you have to have a passport. If you keep carrying it around with you, you could lose it—and then you won't be able to get out of the country, and they wouldn't let you into America even if you did. I could still go by myself, of course, and I just might. So let me have it. You've shown it to everybody you know anyway." He handed it over, but he wasn't happy about it.

When their tickets arrived—paid for by their American hosts—Nkosi wanted to show them around as well. After another round of debate, Gail similarly scotched that idea.

In July 1999 they departed from Johannesburg's damp and dreary winter and, almost sixteen hours later, arrived in New York on a humid summer day. Nkosi was exhausted from the trip and drained by the heat, yet almost deliriously excited as well—and although they were driven straight to a hotel to give them an opportunity to sleep a bit and try to deal with their jet lag, he was impatient to see what there was to be seen. For the next week, as they moved almost constantly about Manhattan, from appearance to appearance, from speech to speech, from interview to interview, he valiantly struggled against his fatigue, only occasionally conceding to Gail that he was the least bit tired. She tried to ration his limited strength, even rescheduled several events to allow him more time to rest, and went so far as to cancel two or three. There was a bit of sightseeing for him on most days, and his neck ached from looking up at buildings taller than anything he had ever seen, but whatever the assignment handed to him, however long the day or however far into the evening it extended, he never let his excitement fade, never once revealed to anyone that his fatigue was catching up with him. Gail thought it was among his most remarkable performances.

"And it was a performance," she later said. "He was onstage almost all the time, meeting people, answering questions from callers on the radio, making little talks at women's clubs and AIDS organizations, at two or three schools. I didn't anticipate before we left that he had already become such a little star in New York—but that's what he was. Of course, that was right down his alley. I think that's actually what kept him going when the going got tough."

Their presence in America provided more than simply a boost to Nkosi's sizable ego. Gail met and came to know a variety of Americans with a genuine interest in the impact of AIDS on Africa. She was also able to raise a small amount of money for Nkosi's Haven and elicit promises for more contributions to come. She told the scores who came to meet her that her plans for HIV-positive women and children in South Africa included several more shelters like the one already open. Moreover, toward the end of their stay in the city a wealthy New Yorker—a woman who would forever remain anonymous—sent word through a third party that she gladly would pay for Nkosi to be given the daily cocktail of antiretroviral drugs that had proved so valuable in treating AIDS victims in America and Western Europe. They were far too expensive for all but the most affluent Africans, among whom Gail certainly did not count herself. On Nkosi's behalf she accepted the woman's generous offer. Even before leaving New York, she telephoned the boy's physician in Johannesburg to tell him the good news.

On the phone that morning, he expressed cautious optimism to her. He reminded her that there was absolutely no cure for AIDS but said that the antiretrovirals—ARVs, as they are known—had enhanced and extended the lives of thousands of HIV-positive men and women and might very well have the same value for Nkosi. In private, with his colleagues who were also treating Nkosi, he worried that it was probably much too late for the boy to reap the full benefits of the medications.

Just once, in his final radio interview, Nkosi acknowledged that his schedule had often been overwhelming. "Sometimes," he said, "when there are thousands and thousands of interviews at once, I get tired—and for five straight days, we had thousands of interviews, on radio and with newspapers and all that. It was a bit too much for me. I didn't get enough energy. I didn't get enough rest." Also, he said, he missed his own bed.

He slept almost the entire way home to Johannesburg— another seventeen-hour trip that took him out across the Atlantic, then down the entire length of Africa. This was Gail's one-word assessment of Nkosi's journey: "heroic."

By the time Gail and Nkosi returned to South Africa, the government was at last talking about AIDS, but it was not speaking the language that pleased her or any of the other physicians, scientists, and activists who had long been lobbying for some affirmative action on the disease.

The new president was Thabo Mbeki. He was the son of one of the ANC's most respected elder statesmen, a man who, like Mandela, had spent years in prison for his active role in the struggle to change his country. Thabo Mbeki had been sent abroad as a young man to be educated in England and in Europe, to be prepared for some influential position of leadership in the ANC and eventually in the multiracial, multicultural South African government envisioned by his father's generation. He had lived in exile for most of his life, a great deal of the time in Zambia, the ANC's headquarters after the apartheid government had outlawed its existence in South Africa. He had returned to his native soil only when Mandela had been released, and he'd been handpicked by Mandela as one of his vice presidents after the 1994 elections.

Five years later, with Mandela's retirement, Mbeki became the second black president of South Africa—and the bane of Gail's existence, as well as that of hundreds of other AIDS activists in the country.

It was a strange turn of events. Mbeki was a handsome, suave, impeccably attired, sophisticated man. He was a knowledgeable and passionate lover of opera. He was fluent in several languages, and he had been one of the chief participants in the long and complicated negotiations between the ANC and the old apartheid apparatchiks following Mandela's release from prison. He was well versed in international jurisprudence and in both African and European history, and he had earned both undergraduate and graduate degrees in economics. There might have been other ANC leaders who considered themselves able successors to Mandela, but none seemed more qualified or better looked the part than Mbeki. He would, it was thought, bring to the presidency a great many gifts that Mandela had lacked—skills in management, contacts in the international diplomatic and economic communities, the energy and enthusiasm of his relative youthfulness, new and innovative ideas for the ongoing process of changing the country from what it had been into what it could be and should be. Mandela was the prophet who had dreamed the dream. Mbeki would be the creative executive who would transform that dream into a lasting reality.

Perhaps he may yet achieve that objective, but almost from the moment of his inauguration in 1999, whatever else he may have done for the people of South Africa has been overshadowed by his peculiar public approach to AIDS. Simply put, what Mbeki said about the disease was that it was not caused by HIV. In fact, he insisted, over and over, that there was no such virus.

SEVEN

For quite some time, with the exception of his mother's funeral in Newcastle, Nkosi had had almost no contact with his biological family—his grandmother, his older sister, his several aunts and uncles—who still lived in Daveyton or just outside in the squatters' settlement of Zenzele. Gail concluded that there was little she could do to change the situation, and she did not mention it to him, nor did he bring it up. With the rush of events in her life and in the boy's—the gradual disintegration of her marriage to Alan, the noisy politics of the new South Africa, the unrelenting urgency of her dream to open not just one but several shelters for infected women and their children, the controversial struggle to enroll Nkosi in school—she did not give the matter much thought or attention.

Even Daphne had stopped coming to see her son as her health had deteriorated in the months before her death. Later

Nkosi would acknowledge that although his memory of his mother was affectionate, it was also a bit fuzzy. "I know I loved my mummy a lot," he told me, "and I know she loved me a lot, but I can't actually remember much about her."

He was similarly vague about Ruth, his grandmother. He once described her to me as being in either her forties or her sixties. He could not be more specific (she and Gail were almost precisely the same age), and he was certain only that she and the other relatives he knew about were black Africans and that they spoke Zulu and Xhosa and "all those other languages like that."

He had by then learned only one language, the English spoken in his foster family, in his suburban neighborhood, and at his school. Although he told his teachers he would be pleased to learn a bit of Zulu, and they did make an effort to teach it to him, over the months he had picked up only a smattering of what would have been his native tongue. To be precise, he knew three Zulu words.

He had this to say about his linguistic limitations: "I would very much enjoy learning to speak my own language, so then I could speak it to my friends. I mean, the friends I have who are black. I also have white friends, and we talk in English, of course. My white friends do not speak Zulu or other black languages like that. But sometimes, when I am walking down the street, black people talk to me in a black language, and I don't know how to talk to them in that language. I always feel embarrassed with myself, and I have to say to them, 'No, I can't speak to you like that because I only speak English.'"

It is not at all surprising that a black child who could remember only living with a white family in a country with such an overwhelming black population would feel some detachment, some itch—however small—to establish some connection with *his* racial family, to have at least some touch—however slight—with his roots. In fact, the suggestion that something was wrong with such an arrangement became an increasingly touchy subject in South Africa, not with specific reference to Nkosi and Gail but to transracial adoptions in general. For several years, even during the apartheid era, couples interested in adopting South African children had flown into Johannesburg and Cape Town from all over the world. Mainly white, they came from America and Western Europe, and they faced very few obstacles, bureaucratic or otherwise. Thousands happily returned to their homes carrying black babies in their arms or with young black children in tow. There were hundreds of transracial adoptions by white South African families as well.

In the latter days of the nineties, however, black voices in the political and academic communities were raised against the practice. Their argument was fairly simple: Black children left without families for whatever reason should be adopted *only* by black families, so as to maintain a connection to their roots and their culture. Otherwise that precious connection would be limited, and eventually it would vanish. There were even a few, including those who should have known better, who condemned transracial adoptions as a grand racist conspiracy devised by the whites of Europe and America and designed to eventually eradicate all traces of original African culture.

Given the history of repression and oppression—after all, Europeans *had* tried in various ways to dilute or destroy

African heritage in their many colonies—these views were perhaps understandable. Yet given that so few black South Africans were economically capable of adding another child to their families—and in fact very few ever did—the opposition to transracial adoptions was a disaster. The call for racial and cultural purity was soon as strident among a few of South Africa's black elite as it had always been among the whites of apartheid. Although there were never any official prohibitions or legal restrictions against transracial adoption, several of its most vocal opponents did ascend to highly influential positions in the new government. Soon the number of black orphans who were adopted by anybody, black or white, began to dwindle. Children's homes and orphanages were overflowing. Even in normal times, that would have been an unfortunate circumstance, but occurring as it did while the number of AIDS orphans was multiplying almost exponentially—and while the new government was saying next to nothing about the virus or the problems it was causing for the country—it was doubly tragic.

Nevertheless, in the context of the country's evolution, it was merely one of countless painful adjustments being made in the new South Africa. Obviously the unofficial discouragement of transracial adoptions failed to meet the minimum standards of any fair-minded democratic nation—that is, doing the most good for the most people. It was also antithetical to the new South Africa's objective of inclusion, of building a multicultural, multiracial society. Whatever its results, it seemed for many to answer a long-stifled urge for racial pride and identity.

For Nkosi, race and roots seemed to be simplistic constructions built on the shaky foundations of how he understood his illness, which he often described as his "funny blood." One afternoon, as we were sitting together in one of the bedrooms at Nkosi's Haven, he reached over, lightly touched the back of my hand, and plaintively said, "Listen to me, Jim. I want to tell you something. I wish that God had made me white. The reason I wish that is because I believe that white children don't get HIV and I think black children do get HIV."

He was right, of course. In South Africa and on the rest of the continent, the virus had rarely infected white babies—but I said nothing.

On another occasion he expressed the same wish to me, though for a different reason. He said if he were white, his color would match that of his foster family. I recall saying something quite feeble to him, something heartfelt and sincere but nevertheless inane. "You know, pal," I said, "everybody should be proud to be whatever color they happen to be, whether it's white like me or black like you or brown or red or white or yellow or even green."

He laughed at the last example. "You mean green like all the snot I produce?" he asked.

I laughed, too.

He also seemed to realize that, given the hand he had been dealt, he had been extraordinarily fortunate to find himself a member of Gail's white tribe. "I think I would rather be living with a white family," he once told me, "because I can eat good food. Every meal I can eat a balanced diet. I don't think I would still be alive if I was all the time eating black-culture food, which I don't mind eating but I believe it is not very good food for me.

"I can remember that my real mummy was actually living in an old shack in the township that had dirty toilets, and I know that with my funny blood I must be living in a clean house with clean toilets."

But he was sensitive enough not to raise or discuss such matters with his grandmother when she began to visit him occasionally in 1999. Nor did he mention them to his aunts and uncles, who often accompanied her, or to his sister, Mbali, who sometimes came along.

Instead he made an honest effort to accept them as family and to make them feel as comfortable as possible when they came. He would give them a tour of the house, would show them the pool and the patio and invite them to swim (no one ever did). He would escort them to his bedroom and identify by name all the stuffed toys that densely populated it. He would point out the autographed poster on his wall of the Grand Prix driver Michael Schumacher. Nearly every time his relatives visited, as though they might have forgotten since their previous call, he would ritualistically introduce them to the dog and the cats, would proudly demonstrate his ever-improving reading skills for them, and with equal pride show them the thick book Mandela had signed and the photograph of himself and Gail with the president. He always kissed and hugged them when they arrived and gave them more enthusiastic hugs when they departed.

Whatever conflicts Nkosi may have entertained about identifying or not identifying with his original culture, about the stark differences between it and the middle-class affluence of his current life, he rarely mentioned them to Gail either, though they did occasionally become the subject of mild debates and disputes in her household. Not that anyone ever considered sending Nkosi to live with his biological family in Daveyton. But Nikki, Gail's bright teenage daughter, could and would sympathetically address the significance of his separation from his roots. "Nkosi really doesn't know his own personal or racial history," she once said, "and because he doesn't, he isn't capable of really socializing or integrating himself with other black Africans. He not only lacks the language, he also lacks the black South African experience. So in that way I don't think that his presence here with us has been an entirely positive thing in his life—and here's why I think that:

"It's very important for him to learn about his own background and about his roots, because they're all a part of who he is, just as my roots and background are a part of who I am. You know, he didn't just suddenly appear from out of the ocean or from under some rock or from behind some tree and attach himself to a white family like us.

"He is a black person. We all know that. It's an undeniable fact. He was born of a black person into a black tribe speaking one of our country's eleven official languages, nine of which are black languages. He is somebody, and he is a specific somebody who came from somewhere, from a specific somewhere, and that somewhere is not our house, this house in this white suburban neighborhood.

"I love him madly, and I always will love him. He is my brother and my friend, but he has a history, and that history is different from my history—and I think he should be educated about his history and should become knowledgeable about it and become proud of it. And when he is, I think he will be a much happier boy."

Whenever this subject arose, Gail would usually nod her philosophical agreement, would not argue that her daughter was wrong (God knows they argued about enough other issues), but she would often assert to Nikki that while the boy might have lost a part or all of his black culture, and perhaps that was unfortunate, it was quite irrelevant because what mattered most was that he was considerably better off exactly where he was. "He has good food and medicine and vitamins and a clean place to sleep and running water that's not only hot if he wants it to be hot—and you know how he likes his hot baths—but also fit to drink and available to him when he wants it," she would argue. "He has a family that loves him completely and respects him and takes care of him and sees to whatever special needs he has, and besides that, he has a lot of friends who feel the same way." Maybe Nkosi did miss his black culture and black roots, she once said to me. "But, quite frankly, I don't know," she added, "because he's never mentioned it to me."

In 1999, after the controversy of his enrollment in school had made Gail and Nkosi relatively famous in the country and his black family had made contact again, tensions had arisen almost immediately. Gail posed no opposition to the resumption of their relationship with the boy after such a long time.

She understood, she said, how difficult the logistics of transportation between Daveyton and Johannesburg were for his
grandmother. The problem, she said, was timing.

"It was just a matter of courtesy," she complained. "The
granny or one of the uncles or aunts would call the house and
announce that they were coming that afternoon or that night
or maybe the next morning, and that they wanted to see Nkosi
or take him with them for the day or back to Daveyton for the
night or the weekend."

The short notice was unacceptable to her, she said. "I expected them to give me ample time to plan and prepare for
their visit or to arrange for Nkosi to go back with them," she
explained. "I had no objection at all to either, but both of us
were very busy. Believe me, it took a hell of a lot of organization to look after him and Nikki, to keep the house going,
to do a little business—precious little—with my company, to
manage the shelter and raise money to keep it alive, not to
mention making plans to open several others.

"Nkosi and I had our own plans and appointments and
schedules. He was spending a lot of time playing the little
prince at the shelter. He had classes and homework and new
friends to see and medical obligations. He also spent time with
Alan, who was very good about maintaining their relationship.
It just wasn't fair of them to expect that, on a couple of hours'
notice, I would drop everything and bust my ass to make them
happy."

It is fair to say that indeed Gail did not "bust her ass" to
make Nkosi's other family happy. "I just couldn't understand
why, for such a long time—for years, in fact—they had been

totally invisible as far as he was concerned and then——bang!——here they are on our doorstep," she said. "There was a complete lack of balance in the relationship. It just went from nothing to a more or less regular interruption of Nkosi's life——and I think it confused him. It certainly confused me."

She was also irritated by Ruth Khumalo's interest in the economic status and financial resources of Nkosi's foster family. "I know it doesn't make me look good to say it, but I have to tell you in all honesty that I deeply resented the fact that they didn't make contact until the two of us had become slightly well known, not to mention that every time his granny came to my house, she would spend a long time explaining again and again that she had no money at all," Gail recalled. "Sometimes I gave her money, sometimes I didn't, but it always struck me that that was the really honest explanation for the sudden resumption of contact between her and her grandson. I know she and her family were desperately poor, and I suppose it's understandable that she couldn't seem to resist the impulse to try to cash in——but to be frank about it, it pissed me off."

Now and then the relationship between them would have its better days, but it would always be edgy and would never much improve. Still, Gail tried not to allow that tension to affect Nkosi's attitude toward his black family. In fact, she said she always referred to them in positive terms in his presence, always concealed from him any hostility or friction she felt, any problem that existed between her and them, said she always encouraged him to respect them and always tried to make clear to him that even though he did not live with them, he was still an important part of them and they were an important part of him. "Didn't your granny look well today?" she would say to him after a visit. Or she would say of his older sister, "Mbali is growing so fast and getting so smart and pretty." Whatever irritation she might have felt, she kept to herself; if she felt compelled to express it verbally, she did so out of his hearing. She understood that, physically and emotionally, Nkosi was a profoundly fragile little boy. What he most required was love and acceptance, hugs and kisses, good times, good food, medicine, and hope. What he definitely did not need in his life was another problem.

But problems unlike any he had ever faced were fast approaching.

We were living our separate lives, Nkosi and I, far apart from one another. In late 1999 he was nearly eleven years old and I was already past sixty. But our orbits were gradually being aligned.

His days were filled with the activities normal for any kid his age—school and homework and fun and games and a few soap operas now and then, with or without Nikki—and also with the burdens and necessities the virus, his funny blood, had placed on him and on Gail.

My own days and nights were consumed by a relentless sequence of ugly and unpleasant assignments that by then had become rather routine for me: war and revolution, famine and flood, death and destruction. They came one after the other, from the Persian Gulf to Mogadishu, from Rwanda to Algeria, from the West Bank to Sarajevo. Any diversion was a blessing. In the autumn of that year, such a blessing arrived in the form of quite an unusual commission.

All throughout 1999, my employer—ABC News—had been heavily focused on elaborate, extensive, and extremely expensive plans for a marathon broadcast on the upcoming New Year's Eve and New Year's Day, grandly marking not only the end of a century but the beginning of the new millennium.

I was living in London then, and had been for several years, but spending what seemed to me to be an inordinate amount of time far from my wife, far from our home, and far from England, on the road in pursuit of stories in most of the rather undesirable venues of Europe, the Middle East, and Africa. Especially Africa. So, although I was slightly taken aback when the producers in New York asked me to report and prepare three or four lengthy stories for the big prime-time millennium broadcast (correspondents like me were rarely included in prime-time programs), I was not at all surprised to be told that those stories should be about and originate in Africa. In addition, I was asked to find an African venue from which I could broadcast live at midnight on the last day of the year. The first choice of my producer, Clark Bentson, was Robben Island, where Nelson Mandela had spent so many years behind bars, and the original plan was for Mandela to be on hand that night to be interviewed by me and, of course, by the ABC anchor, Peter Jennings. Overtures were made to Mandela, and he more or less agreed. The New Yorkers pronounced this a splendid idea, until Bentson estimated the costs—travel, accommodations, camera crews, engineers, satellite transmission, and the like—and presented them with a budget for the project. South Africa quickly disappeared from our agenda.

Bentson, ever resourceful (in my view one of the three or four ablest television producers in the world), began scouring the African map for a country that would provide a suitable and acceptable combination of picture, story, and cost. Eventually, he settled on Djibouti, a tiny and obscure nation situated on the Horn of Africa, on whose inhospitable but starkly beautiful landscape—a moonscape, really—thousands of refugees had settled, trying to escape the chronic combat and chaos of neighboring Somalia and Ethiopia.

Off we went, first to gather the pictures for several stories about politics and wildlife in Africa, about its past and about its future. Our gypsy itinerary included South Africa, Zambia, Malawi, Botswana, Ethiopia, and Uganda, then back to London to write, edit, and package the stories before, late in December, heading to Djibouti for the millennium broadcast.

It was on this long and difficult journey that I finally came to grips with Africa's most significant reality, one that had been staring me in the face for quite some time.

For several years by then, I had been witnessing firsthand AIDS's assault on all the many countries in which I'd worked. I had broadcast several stories about the virus and its effects, had seen hundreds or perhaps thousands of its victims, young and old, had watched a few of them die, had attended some of their funerals—and yet I had not felt the slightest stirring of urgency within me. Looking back now, I believe that in every instance I had been employing the same psychological trick that had served me so well in my coverage of wars. In order to perform the work of the moment, without becoming paralyzed by the horrors of the moment, I would simply shut down emotionally. It was a technique I had mastered, and with only one exception—the massacres in Rwanda in 1994—it had always worked. Perhaps the best and most honest means of expressing this is simply to say that, quite unbelievably, I had willed myself not to become engaged in the story of AIDS in Africa and, as a result, quite incredibly, had not found it all that *interesting.*

Then, in mid-November 1999, on the last leg of our millennium trip, Bentson and I and the camera crew landed in Kampala, the capital of Uganda, to interview its president, Yoweri Museveni. It was then that my attitude began to change.

A tall and powerfully built man who had led the Ugandan military in a successful coup against the infamous Idi Amin, Museveni came equipped with easy answers for all my questions about the future of Africa in general and his country in particular. He struck me as quite a thoughtful man, if also something of a benevolent dictator who believed that the people of Uganda needed to be carefully educated before they would be ready for a full democracy.

We sparred about what I described as his one-party politics. "No, no, no," he said. "You have given Uganda one too many parties. We practice *no-party* politics, and for a while we will continue to do so, until the people are completely prepared for something different, something more."

We left it at that, and I changed the subject. In the stack of research material I'd read on the plane and in my hotel room the night before, I'd noticed statistics listing Uganda as one of only two African nations (the other was Senegal) in which the HIV infection rate had actually turned downward. It had once been among the hardest hit by the virus, with more than 10 percent of its adult population infected. In every other country on the continent, the rate of infection was spiraling exponentially upward at a terrifying pace. Not in Uganda. "So," I asked Museveni, "if no other African government has been able to make such progress, how have you done it?"

His answer would change everything for me. "First," he said in his rumbling basso profundo, "unlike the other governments, my own government has truly and honestly recognized HIV and AIDS as the most dangerous enemy our people have. Second, we have worked night and day for many months, and we have asked for assistance and brought in knowledgeable people to help us devise both offensive and defensive strategies. Third, we are determined that, regardless of how much damage it has already done to us—I mean, regardless of the vast numbers of our citizens it has already killed and the vast numbers who have already been infected and who, we know, will eventually also die—we simply will not—*will not, will not*—allow this virus to continue eating away at our people. We will not allow it to destroy our future as a country."

President Museveni outlined the various components of the strategy: intense and constant public education about the infection's causes, how it is transmitted, and how it can be prevented; the public distribution of millions of condoms, and a national advertising campaign to encourage their use; a mandatory focus on HIV/AIDS at every level of government, from meetings of his ministers and their departments, to the generals in the army, to every police officer in every precinct, to every doctor and every nurse in every hospital and clinic, even down to the eldest of tribal elders in the smallest rural villages; the enlistment and involvement of all nongovernment organizations in the country, including the churches, with constant pressure on those groups reluctant to get involved.

"In other words," Museveni concluded, "AIDS is not only on our national agenda, it is on our minds all the time. In my meetings, when we discuss the economy, imports and exports, anything at all, whatever it is, we do so within the context of AIDS and HIV. When we discuss budgets and taxes, we do so with the understanding that the presence of the virus among us and its threat must be a part of our planning. When the subject is the military, we acknowledge that it is a threat to our national security."

Finally I asked him about all those condoms and the Catholics of Uganda. "Well," he laughed, quite heartily, clearly already savoring what he was about to say, "I'll tell you a little story about that." Approximately a third of the country's 23 million citizens are Catholics, he began, and many of them are influenced by their parish priests, who are in turn influenced by the bishops, who always listen to the archbishop, "who does not listen to anybody, except God, from time to time," the president chuckled. When the program for distributing condoms was announced, and even after it was under way, the archbishop began to protest publicly, to describe it as an un-christian and certainly an un-Catholic enterprise that would encourage premarital sex among young people and violate the church's ban on birth control. Museveni said he listened to the archbishop's condemnations for a few weeks, then summoned him to the presidential compound for a face-to-face meeting.

"And what did you say to him?" I asked.

"Well," said the president, "this is what I said to him. I said to him, 'Your Eminence, shut up!'"

"And did he?"

"He did. He was very angry with me, but he immediately ceased his blathering. He did not like it, and he still does not like it—but I can tell you that he says absolutely nothing about the condoms, not in public at least, and neither do his bishops or priests."

Aha! Something could be done, I thought. And even if it had taken the heavy-handed tactics of a rather fearsome and powerful politician, it *had* been done, and it was working. The number of Ugandans being infected was steadily declining be-cause something had been done. An effort had been made.

It was a revelation to me. Until that moment, never having observed any African government doing anything at all about HIV and AIDS, I'd been thoroughly persuaded that nothing could be done or at least nothing *would* be done to prevent the continued infection of so many millions on the continent. It matched my more general experience in Africa, especially in sub-Saharan Africa, a region of over 600 million people, more than half of whom lived in abject poverty with no access to health care, to sanitation, to clean water, to education, even to their governments, such as they were. I was persuaded that instability, corruption, dictatorial regimes, civil wars, entrenched poverty, rampant crime, squalor, social havoc, chaos, and diseases of all kinds—including AIDS—had transformed the old dreams of freedom and independence from colonialism into a perpetually recurring nightmare. As for the "African Renaissance," whose beginnings President Clinton claimed to have recognized in 1997 and which was the constant theme in the high-flown speeches and writings of South African president Thabo Mbeki, that was, I thought, mere empty rhetoric, disappearing like wisps of smoke from a campfire.

In late 1999 *my* vision of Africa was of a continent in rapid decline, regressing, slipping ever backward into its past. Since I believed that to be the case, I also believed that every story yet to be done—about AIDS or about this plan or that project or this new leader or that new reform—would be precisely the same as the previous one, with only a few names and faces and numbers and places changed here and there. How many times could this same story be broadcast? My pessimism about Africa was inherent in my detachment and my disinterest in the AIDS catastrophe, in my determination to treat it as just another story, broadcast today, forgotten tomorrow.

In Uganda, I discovered I was wrong.

It is difficult for me to admit, but I am truly ashamed that it took such a long time—but at last I was *interested*. What I didn't realize was that precisely because I was interested, the psychological shield on which I had long depended for protection against any uncomfortable and inconvenient emotional investment was about to be penetrated.

W hen the new millennium began, I was where I had been assigned: in Djibouti with Clark Bentson, along with a camera crew and a pair of engineers operating a satellite dish that was beaming pictures to New York from a desolate refugee camp, far out in the middle of nowhere, at the opposite end of Africa from Gail and Nkosi in Johannesburg.

Although an anonymous benefactor in New York had recently begun paying the cost of the antiretroviral cocktail for Nkosi, Gail did not begin the New Year with any great expectations. The medicines, which had been far beyond her means and much too expensive to be donated by Nkosi's doctors (who were already treating him gratis), had enhanced and extended the lives of thousands of HIV-infected patients, and when he'd begun taking it, she was cautiously optimistic. Nevertheless, Gail soon realized that Nkosi was not improving at all. In fact, he was noticeably declining. His speech seemed to grow slightly more slurred with each passing day, and his reserves of energy were more quickly depleted. In December he had agreed to accompany his grandmother, Ruth, on a visit to his mother's grave in Newcastle, but as the day for the trip approached, he seemed less and less interested, and ultimately he declined to go. He told his grandmother on the phone that he was simply too tired.

His doctors finally admitted to Gail that the antiretroviral treatment had probably been initiated too late to be of much benefit to him. Moreover, the medicine seemed to open the way for a return of his diarrhea, and while his weight had been stabilized for quite some time, in December and January the pounds began to slip from his tiny frame. He soon took on the appearance of a cancer patient undergoing chemotherapy. He was losing his hair, and what remained of it had lost its tight curl. "He had the sad face of a little old man," Gail remembered.

Nkosi was well aware of what was happening to his body, understood that the virus was taking full command, that it was no longer just a matter of funny blood, and despite the efforts of Gail and Nikki to keep his spirits up, he was often deeply depressed.

One afternoon early in the year, when he was making a teary fuss about taking his medications, protesting that they tasted bad, that they were causing him to soil his trousers and his bed, Gail asked bluntly if that meant he had decided he wanted to die.

"Do you want to be with your mummy?" she said

He shook his head no.

"Well, all right, then," Gail said. "We've had this discussion before, haven't we?"

He nodded his head yes.

"And you and I, we have a deal, don't we?"

Nkosi said, "Yes, we have a deal. I take my medicine, and—"

"And," Gail finished his sentence, "we fight together. That's our deal. You take your medicine, and both of us fight—and then, if you decide you want to cop out and give up—"

Nkosi interrupted her. "I don't want to cop out," he said. "I don't want to give up."

"Well, then don't. Be as strong as you possibly can."

He was crying again by now. "I can't help it," he said.

She gathered him to her, held him close. "Of course you must cry, my darling," she said. "Of course you must cry."

Remembering that moment, Gail later explained that although it sounded callous of her, although she knew his condition to be terminal, she believed that if she allowed him to think he was dying, he would die. Her goal each day was to buck him up a bit, to keep him in the game. "I had to try to treat him as normally as possible and to maintain his life as normally as possible," she said, "but at the same time, I had to acknowledge his fears and recognize his physical and emotional needs."

Nkosi once asked her, "Mummy Gail, where does AIDS come from?"

She said, "I wish I could give you an answer to that question, darling, but I can't. I just can't—and I can't do anything to change the facts either, no matter how ugly they are. You've got it, and I know you hate it, and I certainly hate it like I've never hated anything in my entire life. But that's the reality."

She did not want him to be frightened of death and always tried to deal straightforwardly with his fears whenever he expressed them, but finally she admitted that she had no idea how to prevent them or even assuage them. "I don't know if there is a right way or not. I talked to child psychologists about it, and they weren't sure there's a best approach to it either. What I always tried to do, I just always tried very hard to make him know that I loved him madly, completely," she said, "and that I would do anything and everything within my power to protect him and keep him safe."

He understood that. At the party celebrating his eleventh birthday in February, he told a local reporter, "The absolutely most important person in my life is my mummy, Gail Johnson, and the second most important person in my life is Nikki Nikki's my big sister—and I really love my doggie, Dukie Boy, and the kitties. I'm really lucky to be living with Mummy Gail, because if I wasn't living with her, I wouldn't be here. I wouldn't—I wouldn't be having the treatment and love."

That was true for Nkosi, of course, but love and treatment were in scarce supply for the other 4 million AIDS victims in South Africa.

Nelson Mandela's retirement from the South African presidency in the previous spring had been celebrated as nothing less than the twilight of a god, the passing of a giant. From around the world came thousands of messages of gratitude for his life, of unbridled praise and adulation for his work. For weeks before and after he left office, he was lavishly feted and toasted as his nation's incomparable savior, an international hero, a living embodiment of extraordinary courage. Few men of any color in any country had ever been accorded such lavish valedictories, and few had so deserved them.

Nevertheless, for Thabo Mbeki, the South Africa inherited from Mandela was no bargain. Crime was rampant all across the country. The murder rate was four times that of the United States—about 25,000 deaths a year, or around 70 every day—but with only 3,500 convictions. In fact, few crimes of any kind were being solved, and a third of all cases were cleared simply by withdrawal of the charges.

Johannesburg, the country's largest city—the financial, cultural, and commercial powerhouse of South Africa—had deteriorated into one of the most dangerous places in the world, its central business district a cardboard city, with hawkers, the homeless, thugs, muggers, pickpockets, and gangsters cramming the streets and jamming the sidewalks. Most of the old shops, restaurants, and businesses had relocated to the northern suburbs, the stock exchange included. Only the municipal and provincial judiciary remained, but lawyers with business in its complex drove from the suburbs directly into well-guarded parking garages that provided access to their offices and the courts without making it necessary for them to go outside, beyond the protective cocoon.

In the principal cities—Johannesburg, Cape Town, Durban—nearly everyone either had been burglarized, carjacked, or mugged or knew someone who had. Nationally, an average of one rape occurred every minute of every hour of every day, the highest rate in the world. This statistic included a horrifying number of sexual assaults on children, even infants—the grim product of a widespread belief that having sex with a virgin would somehow either protect a man from the HIV virus or remove it from his body.

In the five years of a black-majority government, at least 250,000 and perhaps as many as 500,000 white South Africans had left the country, most of them from the professional class, many of them citing crime as the reason for their departure. One survey that appeared just as Mbeki was taking over suggested that three out of four of the white professionals who still remained in the country were seriously considering emigration, citing not only crime and public safety but also the quality of education available to their children and the government's affirmative-action programs in which blacks were getting jobs in preference to whites. And yet 40 percent of blacks were unemployed, and 70 percent lived below the official poverty line, 7 million of them in the squalor of shantytowns.

With all this, as well as a still-struggling economy, Mbeki faced a daunting task. Business confidence was lagging. Foreign investors were wary, reluctant to risk their money in a country plagued by such enormous and seemingly intractable problems.

And then, of course, there was AIDS. Adding to the 4 million people already living—and dying—with the virus, there were 1,700 new infections every day. One in five pregnant women was HIV-positive, and on average more than half of them would infect their babies. More than 70,000 infants were born HIV-positive each year, and 7,000 babies died of AIDS each month. Half of South Africa's boys who were then fifteen would not live to see thirty, and 20 percent of all young girls, from ages thirteen through nineteen, were infected. Yet for some months in the early part of his tenure, President Mbeki had nothing to say about a scourge that was clearly jeopardizing the future of his country.

When he finally did address the subject, he immediately ignited a firestorm of controversy. On one occasion he declared publicly that the virus HIV did not cause AIDS. In other remarks he cast doubt on the very existence of the virus. In still another venue, he said that perhaps it did exist but no one was certain, and even if it did, no one was sure it was the cause of AIDS. The real causes, he insisted, were poverty and an unhealthy diet.

Doctors, scientists, epidemiologists, microbiologists, AIDS activists, and editorial writers both in South Africa and in countries beyond its borders responded furiously. Some of their most prominent leaders demanded a meeting with the president, an opportunity to discuss his views, to compare them with the findings of the world's medical-research community, to demonstrate to him the error of his ways. All such entreaties were rejected. There would be no meeting. The president had made up his mind, and there he would stand. He knew what he knew. He was castigated, criticized, and lampooned—but his heels were firmly dug in, and he would not be moved.

There was considerable speculation about the source of Mbeki's absurd ideas, and eventually the consensus was that he must have absorbed his misinformation from the Internet. He would not say.

His official response to the furor was to appoint a National AIDS Council, but he excluded from its membership anyone who disagreed with his own thesis, including all the country's most important medical experts, researchers, and representatives of nongovernmental organizations working with AIDS victims. Those he named to it took a benign, know-nothing position and vowed to get to the bottom of what was causing the deaths of so many thousands of South Africans. If there was an answer, they swore, they would find it.

It would have been laughable if it wasn't so tragic. Mbeki's views were being accepted and echoed with such fervent fealty throughout his ANC bureaucracy that in official circles they became pure gospel. The patently silly and thoroughly irrelevant AIDS council was the extent of his government's AIDS policy. In reality there *was* no policy. In reality nothing was being done.

Mbeki was under siege. Reporters and correspondents granted interviews with him—they were few and far between —were instructed by his press secretary, Parks Mankahlana, *not* to ask questions about you-know-what. When one journalist ignored the prohibition and did ask, the president simply puffed on his pipe and stared silently into the distance.

Given all that, it is fairly reasonable to assume that when Mbeki was informed that the 13th International Conference on AIDS would be held in Durban in July 2000, he was probably not all that pleased, even though he was asked to be its keynote speaker, and even though its 11,000 participants from 178 countries would be spending a considerable chunk of money in his own country. He would be even less pleased when it was over.

EIGHT

I had become, by then, my network's informal AIDS-in-Africa correspondent. I lacked official portfolio or credentials, but I began nevertheless to push for and promote stories about the virus and its devastating effect on all the sub-Saharan countries—the serious threat it posed to their economies and their armies, its impact on their fragile infrastructures, and the policy or absence of policy of their governments. Perhaps my bosses were merely indulging me, but whatever their reasons, they were both cooperative and, to a degree, themselves interested. Although their passion was clearly not as intense as mine—in terms of foreign news, they had several other fish to fry, and I often thought I heard just a note of weary condescension in their voices from across the Atlantic—I did not expect it to be. It was quite enough that they gave me considerable leeway in planning a series of assignments that focused on the disease. More important, they bankrolled the stories.

So in February, on a typically drab and dreary London morning, when Clark Bentson dropped a copy of the press release about that summer's International AIDS Conference on my desk, I immediately penciled in the dates on my calendar and began mapping out our basic strategy not only for being in South Africa when the conference took place but also for convincing the producers in New York that it was a worthwhile assignment. In those days, even before the terrorist attacks, budgets at all the network news divisions were excruciatingly tight, and African stories were frightfully expensive. To their everlasting credit, however, the ABC executives whose hands were on the broadcast purse strings were usually amenable to our ideas, as long as we displayed some reasonable sensitivity to their own financial pressures and constraints. Their answer on the AIDS conference was positive, though, as was generally the case, they asked that the coverage be combined with several other stories so as to amortize and reduce the costs-per-story.

"How about Nkosi?" Bentson suggested.

"What's that?" I asked.

"You know, the kid."

"Oh, yeah," I said.

The specific name had faded from my memory, but I had by then heard of a black child in Johannesburg and his white foster mother who had somehow managed to put a human face on AIDS in South Africa. In fact, almost anyone with any interest at all in AIDS or in Africa in general or South Africa in particular would have been aware of them. Still, my knowledge of exactly who they were and what they had done was sketchy at best.

"Read this," Bentson said, handing over a sheaf of stories about them. I did. The boy was immediately put on our list, though I must admit he was not at the top of it. I'd already broadcast several stories about children with AIDS (Kebo included), and another one didn't strike me as an awfully urgent priority. The fact that in the former bastion of apartheid, this boy was living with a white family was intriguing, but not enough to bump him ahead in the lineup.

It was only when Bentson later informed me that Nkosi was scheduled to be one of the keynote speakers in the opening session of the AIDS conference—along with the president of South Africa, Thabo Mbeki, that I thought, Bingo!

Just as she had been quite uncertain about the advisability of taking Nkosi to New York, Gail was not quickly convinced that it was a good idea for him to appear at the conference. She did not immediately tell him about the invitation. Knowing him, she thought he would probably want to do it, and she wanted to give herself time to carefully weigh all the factors.

The trip to Durban would not present much of a problem. The flight from Johannesburg was a very brief one. The real problem was that she could now measure the incremental decline of the boy's health almost by the hour, could see that his daily reserves of energy were rapidly dwindling and were usually depleted by noon. She noticed that the only pleasure he seemed to be deriving from his life was in the increasing amount of time he was spending at the shelter. It was very difficult for her to watch this steady and inexorable deterioration. He had consistently been, by nature, a jovial and joyous child. Despite everything that had happened to him, there had always seemed to be a delicious grin on his face or at least lurking mischievously around the corner. Laughter had come so easily to him. But by now, however, only glimpses of that beloved personality remained.

Having seen his most recent blood-test results, Gail knew what was happening to him. His CD4 count was terrifying. CD4s are white blood cells that play a significant role in the human body's immune system and response, and their number is a clear indication of a patient's condition. More than any other type of cell, HIV targets CD4s, and without medication to counter it, it will relentlessly attack and destroy more and more of them, causing a drastic reduction in the count, usually by about 30 to 100 per year in most HIV-positive people. A normal CD4 count is approximately 600 to 1,500 cells. As the count diminishes, the person is more vulnerable to opportunistic infections, and it is those infections (toxoplasmosis, tuberculosis, Pneumocystis pneumonia, and HIV nephropathy, a kidney disease) that are responsible for most AIDS deaths.

In many cases antiretroviral drugs can successfully reverse or stop the reduction of CD4s, producing what is known as the "Lazarus effect," when a patient moves quickly from death's door back to work within three months. There is no cure for AIDS, but the antiretrovirals can help keep the worst symptoms at bay for a sustained period of time. In Nkosi's case, however, as his doctors had told Gail, the infection had already progressed much too far for the medicines to be of any help to him.

For example, in September 1998, his CD4 count had been only 13. By the time he returned from New York not quite two years later, it was down to 2.

Gail realized that it was only a matter of time—and that raised questions for her about even telling the boy that he'd been invited to speak at the world's most important and prestigious AIDS gathering. For her the most salient of those questions was, was it fair to him?

On the other hand, the prospect of putting him on the same stage with the South African president was awfully tempting. Mbeki had become the archenemy of every AIDS activist in the country, including Charlene Smith. A columnist for the *Mail & Guardian* and a most formidable woman, she had cheekily described Mbeki as the country's "chief undertaker." As acerbic as that description may have been, it was mild in comparison with others offered by those who found Mbeki's continuing public posture and rhetoric on AIDS and HIV to be downright bizarre, if not murderous.

Mbeki had undergone some mysterious transformation. Several years earlier, as South Africa's vice president, he had said, "For too long we have closed our eyes as a nation, hoping the truth was not so real. For many years we have allowed the HIV virus to spread . . . and now we face the danger that half of our youth will not reach adulthood. Their education will be wasted. The economy will shrink. There will be a large

number of sick people whom the healthy will not be able
to maintain. Our dreams as a people will be shattered." No
one in the government had nailed it any better than that.
Yet since he was president, his statements had grown increasingly weird. He had alleged that an "omnipotent apparatus"
was using the disease as an instrument of genocide against
black Africans. He had said this "apparatus" was promoting
conventional views to denigrate black Africans, to profit from
their misery, and ultimately to destroy them. Among the
instruments of this fiendish "apparatus" he had uncovered
were pharmaceutical companies, scientists, physicians, medical researchers, and Western governments. He had once even
hinted that the CIA was involved, either directly or periph-
erally, though he admitted he was not certain which. Eventually, referring specifically to Nkosi, he said the boy was
gradually being poisoned by the antiretroviral medications he
was receiving.

About the only time Mbeki ever ventured even into the
general neighborhood of the truth was when he described
poverty as the cause of the widespread collapse of the human
immune system in Africa. Certainly the AIDS pandemic on the
continent does not exist in a vacuum. Clearly its effects are
greatly multiplied and exacerbated by famine, poor hygiene,
poor education, and poor infrastructure. In other words, by
poverty. Yet poverty is only an aider and an abettor, a facilita-
tor of the virus, not a cause of the disease. Nkosi's surprising
longevity, for example, was certainly due in part to the diet
and hygiene that were a part of his life with Gail and her fam-

ily, but their absence in his infancy had not infected him. His
mother had transmitted the virus to him. It was as simple and
as sad as that.

President Mbeki, though—for whatever his reasons—was
persuaded otherwise, and that would have grievous consequences for his country. For example, two drugs—AZT and
nevirapine, both endorsed by the World Health Organization
had been shown to lessen dramatically the odds of mother-to-
child transmission of the virus, exactly the manner in which
Nkosi had been infected. A single dose of nevirapine given to an
HIV-positive mother during her labor and one dose given to her
baby soon after its birth reduced the chances of transmission by
50 percent. These medicines were widely available by then to
patients in the wealthier nations of the world, but not in those
hardest hit by AIDS, including South Africa. Eventually the
pharmaceutical companies came under enormous pressure to
reduce the prices of their products, to make them more available in the developing world. One of the companies that manu-
factured nevirapine had responded by offering it in large
quantities to South Africa without charge. They waited, ready
and willing to ship the drug to the country where nearly 200
newborns were being infected by their mothers every day. For
months they heard nothing from Mbeki's government. Finally it
formally and publicly refused the company's offer, explaining
that nevirapine was untested and dangerous. Neither was
true—but Mbeki knew what he knew.

Archbishop Desmond Tutu, the Nobel laureate, was
shocked. "The government's stand on nevirapine," he thun-
dered, "has made South Africa the laughingstock of the world."

Mandela, the former president, said nothing. Nothing in public, at least. His friends said he was in an awfully tricky and difficult position. He did not disagree with Tutu regarding the government's policies on AIDS and AIDS medications, but at the same time he did not wish to be seen as interfering with Mbeki's stewardship of the country.

AZT was already available at several private clinics and hospitals in the country, but the government issued a national ban on its use by doctors, prohibiting them from prescribing it for HIV-positive patients, including pregnant women, in public medical facilities. The reason given? AZT was untested and dangerous. Again, neither charge was true —but Mbeki knew what he knew.

The president, Gail and other activists decided, had to be challenged again and again—and who better to pose that challenge than a frail and fragile kid who was dying from the infection of a virus whose very existence Mbeki questioned? She asked Nkosi if he'd like to make the speech of his life.

His eyes lit up.

W e are all the same," he was saying in that soft, singsong soprano. There he was, out in the scruffy garden beside the shelter that bore his name, practicing his speech—and there I was, hidden in the shrubbery, eavesdropping, spying, watching and listening, amazed, captivated.

Inside Nkosi's Haven, I met Gail. She was being supremely warm and cooperative, lending a helping hand to the camera crew and Bentson as they rearranged furniture, dragging an old easy chair first here, then there, replacing it with a couch, shifting tables and lamps, opening and closing the drapes to measure the difference in available light, snaking electrical cables through the rooms, setting up light stands, generally lending an air of disarray and confusion to a house already jammed with screaming babies and noisy children. As she assisted in the preparations for our shoot, Gail would often stop to wipe a nose or change a diaper or transfer one baby from a high chair into an infant seat or referee a dispute between a couple of the older kids—and in between she would pause for a quick, quiet chat with one of the mothers, most of whom appeared frightened of or at least a bit uncomfortable with the transformation of their home into a television set.

At one point, when the chaos seemed to have reached a breaking point, Gail marched to the center of the cluttered parlor and, clapping her hands, tried to get everyone's attention.

"People!" she shouted to the children. "People, we have to have some order in here! Otherwise, you will all be killed!"

The noise abated momentarily, and the older children, giggling at her threat, watched her.

"Now, children, these are our new friends," she said, spreading her arms to indicate the four white strangers who had invaded their home. "They are very nice men, and you will like them. I repeat, you *will* like them. Now, behave yourselves, and remember what I told you this morning."

She smiled.

"Do not," she said, "I repeat, do not ask them for money until *after* they're finished."

She paused again.

"Now, where the hell is 'Kosi?" she said.

She seemed slightly surprised when I told her I had seen him in the garden, rehearsing his speech.

"I'll tell you the truth," she said. "I love him dearly, but he drives me to drink."

In that first encounter, she struck me as a woman with too much to do and not enough time to do it, a bundle of open nerves, frazzled and occasionally frantic—and yet, in her own unorthodox way, totally organized and utterly self-disciplined. As I would soon learn, whatever her objectives happened to be, long term and short, she was always moving in their general direction. Her specific goal that afternoon was to open Nkosi's Haven to a network television crew from America and thereby introduce it and its namesake to millions of viewers in the United States. She knew a good story when she saw it. So did I.

She called Nkosi in from the garden, and he entered the house with that smile on his face—a smile that brightened my life and still lingers in my memory.

"I'm Jim," I said, shaking his tiny hand.

"You can call me Nkosi," he replied.

"I saw you out there."

"Yes, I know," he said. "I saw you, too."

"May I read your speech?" I asked.

"I wrote it myself," he said, handing over the sheets of paper.

We sat down together at a table already crowded with children either eating their lunches or throwing them at each other. When I had finished reading his remarks, I told him how impressed I was. "It's very good," I said.

"I think so, too," he said.

"And you wrote this all by yourself?"

"Every word," he said, "but Mummy Gail typed it on the computer and printed it for me."

"So Mummy Gail is your secretary," I joshed.

He smiled again. "Sort of," he said.

I began to explain why we were there, what we were doing, what would be happening, what his part in it would be. "You shouldn't be nervous," I counseled. "I think it might even turn out to be fun."

He grinned. "I'm not nervous," he said, "and almost all the time, I have fun. Mummy Gail says maybe I have *too* much fun."

I said, "Well, Mummy Gail is wrong."

She heard my comment and stuck her head around the corner from the kitchen.

"Mummy Gail is wrong," I continued, undaunted, raising my voice a bit to make certain she could hear. "You can never be too rich or have too much fun."

She smiled only slightly and disappeared, but Nkosi's grin expanded to fill his face. Looking back, I think it was that grin that got me.

The rest of the afternoon went as smoothly as could be expected for a three-ring circus with a cast of ten mothers and fifteen children. We were introduced to the kids by Gail, who identified them by the nicknames she had given them: The Screamer, The Terminator, The Hulk, and Weepy Willie. There were sit-down interviews with Gail alone and Nkosi alone, then Gail and Nkosi together, then with some of the children in the shelter, then with Nkosi and the children, then with two or three of the mothers, all of whom seemed absolutely genuine in their gratitude to Gail and their praise for her work and her compassion.

A mother named Grace said that after her husband had died of AIDS, though not before infecting her, she had lived with her in-laws, including a brother-in-law who had tried repeatedly to engage her in sex. "So I decided to take my three children and leave," she said, "and for three months, I think, we had no place to stay. We just lived on the street, and we ate garbage—and then I heard of Nkosi's Haven." She smiled and sighed. "Now we all have a home."

The others told much the same story.

Feroza Mohammed and her six-year-old son, Ismail, were living in a squatters' camp near Johannesburg when they heard about Nkosi's Haven in December 1999. She had no parents, and because she had AIDS, she had been shunned by her husband's Muslim family, although he was the one who had infected her. They made her leave their home, she said, even though she was pregnant. "I came here," she said, "because there was no other place." Her baby—whom everyone called Mickey—was born in June but died soon afterward. "I wish I could fight," Feroza said, "but I am so tired of fighting."

Mpho Mavusa, already drawn and gaunt, had arrived in February. "Miss Gail is a wonderful, wonderful woman," she said. "She is not afraid of us because we have the AIDS. She even gives us hugs and kisses us, and when we have the diarrhea, you know, she is not afraid to help us clean ourselves."

I had read similar stories of Gail's compassion, including an account by the *Mail & Guardian* columnist Charlene Smith, who had written that when she and Gail had been nominees for a prestigious women's award in 1999, they had met a black woman—also a nominee and HIV-positive—from a distant suburb of Johannesburg who was struggling not only to survive but also to keep her family intact. Gail had not forgotten her, had organized assistance and aid for her, had visited her repeatedly, despite the distance and all her other responsibilities, and had helped her achieve some stability in her life and in her children's lives.

I mentioned that to Gail, and she shrugged. "Whatever I can do, I try to do," she said. "Sometimes I try to do things I can't do, and sometimes I know I probably can't do them even before I try—but you never *really* know until you try."

I asked her about her early days with Nkosi. "He couldn't speak a word of English," she recalled, "and he was just such a tiny little guy and very special—and when I took him home, he grew on us. He adjusted so beautifully. He was contagious, so to speak.

"Of course, he had infections in his adenoids, his throat, his ears—so he was quite a messy child. His glands were swollen, he had tuberculosis, and he had thrush, which meant it was very hard for him to swallow, and he produced mountains of mucus. Mountains of mucus! Most of the time, he looked like a glazed doughnut.

"If someone had told me a few years ago that I would have a black child with AIDS in my family, in my home, I would have thought they were absolutely insane. But I've got him, and it hasn't all been a Sunday picnic, but I don't regret one moment

of it, because he has made me and my family better people. It
has been absolutely marvelous."

I asked if, in those early days, she had told friends and
others of Nkosi's condition.

"Yes, I did," she said. "I went public with him immediately,
because that's an important issue, as far as I'm concerned. I
would prefer that people who have HIV/AIDS disclose that
they do so that they can be treated, so that they can be helped.
But I also told people about Nkosi's condition because I thought
it was necessary to reassure people and members of the public
that you can actually care for someone who's infected and not
be infected yourself."

I asked her if she'd do it again.

"If I was younger, yes, I suppose I would, because I doubt
very much whether I would have been involved with AIDS to
the extent that I am if I hadn't found Nkosi—or if his mother
hadn't found me. I was in the public-relations business, and
then the brother of a friend of mine died from an AIDS-related
disease, and that's when I got involved. I helped open another
care center, which closed because we ran out of money,
and that's where I first met Nkosi—his mother brought him
there—and that's where I took him home from. But if Nkosi
had not survived, I mean, if he had died as an infant, as most
HIV-positive babies do, I don't think I would have done what
I've done. I don't know. He's been a real little motivator. He
kick-started me."

I asked if she was satisfied with what she'd done so far, that
is, creating Nkosi's Haven.

"Well, yes," she said, "but it's nowhere near enough. Now

that we've got this house, I intend on having a hell of a lot more. I want to open a sort of national franchise or chain of them. It's terribly important."

When I interviewed Nkosi, I began with fairly harmless questions, learned that his favorite foods were pizza and hamburgers and roast chicken, that his favorite soccer club was the Kaizer Chiefs, that his favorite leisure activity was taking hot baths, sometimes with Gail in her big tub, but most of the time by himself.

"I just love to stay there for a long time, maybe for hours if Mummy Gail will let me," he said. "I like to take baths here [at Nkosi's Haven] because nobody tells me it's time to get out. They just let me stay as long as I want. I ask them to fill the tub really high, and then I try to float in the water. Do you ever do that, Jim?"

"Listen, kid," I said, "I'm asking the questions here."

He laughed.

I asked him about school.

"Oh, I love it," he said. "I'm a very good boy. I love my teachers, and my teachers love me." He paused. "I think they do," he added.

"I know that some of the children were worried at first, you know, when I first went to school, that they would get AIDS from me," he said, "but some of the other kids told them, 'Nkosi is a gentle little boy. He will not harm you.'"

When I sensed that he was getting tired, I suggested that perhaps we should finish up.

"You haven't asked me about death," he said.

"No, I haven't," I replied. "Do you want to talk about it?"

"I know about death, yes. I've thought about it. I can talk about it. You should ask me about it."

And so I did.

"I feel like I'm going to die pretty soon, like my mother died," he said. "Very soon, I think. But at least she got to be a grown-up. I don't think I will ever be a grown-up. I just hope this cocktail helps very soon. I can't feel happy. I don't know.

"I think heaven will be a really nice place. I think I will be a handsome guy in heaven, and also I will see my mother. I think we will dance together."

A couple of tears escaped his eyes and ran in a narrow silver stream down his cheeks.

"Okay," I said to him and to the crew, "that's it."

But he shook his head.

"No, no, no," he said.

"I hate having this disease," he continued, "and I wish so much it would just go away so I don't have to be sick and have diarrhea. I pray to God every night that it will go away. But I know it won't.

"I wish I could be well like my sister is. My sister's name is Mbali, and she is not sick at all. It makes me think of my mother. Her name was Daphne, and she died with the HIV. But my mummy Gail, she said, 'Don't even think about it. Don't think about death. Just think about what's ahead of you. You've still got a long life and lots more things to do.'"

There were a few tears elsewhere in the room. We were finished.

The next day I came back to see him at the shelter, listened as he read some stories to me and to the children. It was obvious that they thought the world of him and just as obvious that he was lapping it up. The day after that, I visited him at Gail's house. We sat and talked with no cameras or microphones. We watched *The Young and the Restless*. I asked him if he wanted me to help him with his speech. He declined.

"Thank you, but Mummy Gail says it has to be only my words, not anybody else's," he said. We took a bit of a walk around the neighborhood. We had a bite to eat.

"Good luck in Durban," I told him as I was going out to my rental car.

"You forgot to say good-bye to Duke," he said.

I said good-bye to the dog and gave him a farewell scratch.

"You forgot the hug," he said.

Nkosi felt so tiny within my arms I felt I might break him in two, yet I was reluctant to release him. And I thought that whatever it was the kid had that was generating all his courage, all his grit and spunk, I wanted a couple of cases.

Of all South Africa's provinces, KwaZulu-Natal, with Durban as its principal city, had been the hardest hit by AIDS. It was the center of the country's raging epidemic. The statistics that seemed so shocking elsewhere were even more astonishing there—but what was most astounding to me was how some of the Zulu women were desperately trying to turn the tide.

The day before the AIDS conference began, we drove out to a rural village to film, of all things, an afternoon of chastity tests. The venue was a soccer field, and by noon a long line of young Zulu women, most of them with their breasts bared, were waiting. They were there to undergo what had once been a standard ritual in their tribal communities when brides-to-be were examined to confirm their virginity, thereby increasing the value of their dowries.

One by one the girls were escorted to small groups of older women, who instructed them to lie down on their backs and open their legs.

Blankets were held up to provide at least some privacy.

When the examination concluded, there were whoops all around, and if the women believed virginity had been confirmed, the girl was given a small ribbon. After a thousand such tests, which stretched through the entire afternoon, the woman who had organized the event declined to say how many girls had not received the ribbons. In other words, how many non-virgins had been discovered.

"Were there any?" I asked.

She would not say.

I asked her if she didn't feel the whole process was intrusive, a violation of the girls' privacy. She said they were under no obligation to be there, that they had come to be tested of their own accord.

Beatrice Ngcobo, the commissioner of the South African Gender and Equality Board, begged to differ.

"Not only is there the issue of privacy and the issue of intrusiveness," she said, "there is also the matter of dignity and respect and freedom of choice—and there is the issue of confidentiality. We have been told, even by some of the girls, that the one who is identified as not being a virgin anymore is often

shunned and ostracized by her friends and by her peers. Even
if she cleanses herself with the slaughter of a goat or some other
ritual, she is still set apart—and we believe that is wrong."

I agreed with her, of course, but I couldn't help thinking as
I left the soccer field that day that at least these women were
trying—trying to do something, however meaningless or
wrongheaded some outsider might choose to regard it. Their
methods would have little effect on the continuing spread of
the virus, but they could at least say to themselves that an effort had been made—and that was something the president of
South Africa could not say.

In Durban the next morning, at the convention center, I
spoke with Dr. Peter Piot, who runs UNAIDS, the principal
United Nations organization dealing with the epidemic world-
wide. We bantered for a few minutes about generalities before
I asked him about Mbeki and his views.

"Our position at UNAIDS is very clear," he replied. "Having a debate today on the cause of AIDS is a waste of time. That
debate should be in the dustbin of history."

But it wasn't. In fact, as the thousands of delegates to the
conference began gathering, Mbeki and his bizarre take on the
origins of the disease were the hot topic du jour.

All manner of supposition was making the rounds: Perhaps
someone in Mbeki's family was infected, and he was simply in
a state of self-defensive denial. Maybe Mbeki himself was infected and simply could not face the fact of his illness. Or
could it be (this was the most malicious) that his decision to

deny medication to infected South Africans, most of whom were poor, was simply his way of removing their burdensome drain on the country's financial resources? That night, in a huge soccer stadium in downtown Durban, these theories and more were passed from delegate to delegate.

The opening ceremonies, broadcast live around the world on satellite, were elaborately staged as a colorful and noisy African tableau, with music and dancers and drummers in traditional costumes on stage, even suspended in the air. Behind a huge chorus of singers was a backdrop of projected images of children with AIDS. There were fireworks and fog machines—and at last there was Thabo Mbeki.

He was not warmly received, especially when he called on scientists and medical researchers to have "sufficient tolerance to respect everybody's point of view." People in the audience of nearly thirty thousand, including thousands who were HIV positive, jeered and booed. "That has nothing to do with our lives!" they shouted.

He continued, unfazed. "Some in our world consider the questions I and the rest of our government have raised around the HIV/AIDS issues . . . as akin to grave criminal and genocidal misconduct," Mbeki said. "What I hear being said repeatedly, stridently, angrily, is, Do not ask any questions.

"I believe that we should speak to one another honestly and frankly, with sufficient tolerance to respect everybody's point of view, with sufficient tolerance to allow all voices to be heard."

Using a familiar rhetorical device, he insisted that all the miseries of Africa should not be blamed on a single virus. It was, of course, a defense against an unmade charge. No one had ever suggested that Africa's myriad problems—poverty, famine, and hunger and the multitude of others—were the product of HIV.

When Mbeki concluded his remarks, there was only a smattering of polite applause, mixed with a number of cat-calls. He seemed unperturbed and, in fact, smiled thinly as he returned to his seat in the front row of chairs arranged on the field. Sitting next to him was his wife, Zanelle. Next to her was Nkosi.

He looked quite spiffy that night in a new blazer and tie, especially tailored to fit his vanishing body, and when he was introduced to a thunderous ovation, he seemed for all the world to be a little boy lost. As he stood in the blinding spotlight and was given a hand mike for his speech, his nervousness was evident. Gail was not far away, seated on the ground below him. She could see him quite clearly, but the glare of the lights on him made it impossible for him to see her. There was a brief, awkward pause—and then came that smile.

"Hi," he said, holding the mike close to his mouth, his words reverberating around the stadium and out into the night. "My name is Nkosi Johnson." Another roar of approval from the crowd was followed by sustained applause. "I live in Johannesburg, South Africa. I am eleven years old, and I have full-blown AIDS. I was born HIV-positive."

In his other hand, he held a copy of his speech, and from time to time he referred to it. Yet for the most part he spoke from memory. He told the vast crowd about his mother's death and her funeral.

"I saw my mommy in the coffin, and I saw her eyes were closed," he said, "and then I saw them lowering her into the ground, and then they covered her up.

"Ever since the funeral, I have been missing my mommy lots, and I wish she was with me, but I know she is in heaven— and she is on my shoulder watching over me, and in my heart."

The crowd was hushed, absorbing every word.

"I hate having AIDS," he continued, "because I get very sick, and I get very sad when I think of all the other children and babies that are sick with AIDS.

"I just wish that the government can start giving AZT to pregnant HIV mothers to help stop the virus being passed on to their babies."

The stadium erupted with wild applause, and the thousands in the audience rose to their feet. Most were unaware that in the moments just after Nkosi had told the crowd his name, Thabo Mbeki had disappeared. His chair was empty.

He did not hear the boy's summation, the lines with which I was already familiar.

"We are all the same."

Smile.

"We are not different from one another."

Smile.

"We all belong to one family."

Smile.

"We love and we laugh, we hurt and we cry, we live and we die."

Then he ended with words I had not heard him rehearse that day.

"Care for us and accept us. We are all human beings. We are normal. We have hands. We have feet. We can walk, we can talk—and we have needs just like everyone else. Don't be afraid of us.

"We are all the same."

There was a heartbeat or two of silence in the stadium, then a tumultuous roar.

Gail was on her feet, bursting with pride, clapping, crying. Her boy had done all that was expected of him, and more.

NINE

As the fight to enroll Nkosi in school had vaulted him and Gail into prominence, his appearance at the AIDS conference had made them even better known in South Africa. And in the squalid settlement outside Daveyton, Ruth Khumalo was beginning to fume to the reporters who came sniffing around for more background on the country's newest hero.

His grandmother and his sister had last seen the boy a couple of weeks before his trip to New York, and both could tell, as anyone could, that he was not doing well at all. Ruth said she knew exactly why. It was because he wasn't getting the love and care that he deserved, she said, and only his family—she and the rest of his *real* family—could provide that.

To one journalist she said she was quite angry, that it wasn't right after all that a black child like Nkosi—a Zulu boy like Nkosi—should be living with a white woman "It is not the way it should be," she complained. To another reporter she offered her own version of how Nkosi had come to leave her daughter's care and become a member of the Johnson household. "Before the clinic closed"—apparently referring to the Guest House—"comes Gail to my daughter," Ruth said. "She talk to my daughter. She say, 'Okay, I can help you, Daphne. I can take this baby, because he is sick.' Or something like that, okay? And my daughter is young, you know, so when she is young, she wants to be free, and she say to Gail, 'Okay.' So Gail takes the baby, and the baby becomes hers—but he should not be with her. He should be always with me."

Either she did not know that her daughter had been terminally ill with AIDS, did not understand that AIDS had killed her, or she was simply ignoring what she knew to be true. Moreover, in those interviews, for the first time—nearly ten years after Nkosi had been handed over by his mother—Ruth raised the specter of exploitation.

"Gail's making money," Ruth said. "I want to tell you, she is making money. She phone, she write, something like that all the time. She is clever. Gail knows that she get something with Nkosi."

When the stories appeared, Gail's response was muted, not at all what I would have expected from her. She said quite simply that both her personal bank account and the books for Nkosi's Haven were open for anyone to examine, including any reporter who wished to do so. A few took her up on it and, finding no discrepancies (a couple were surprised at her limited means), saw no reason to believe that she was using the boy as a means of earning money. Gail was not on the edge of poverty, but she was a single mother with very modest assets. She had, in fact, shut down her public-relations business and invested almost everything she had—beyond the funds she needed for keeping her house and for raising Nkosi and Nikki—in the shelter and in plans for expanding the concept into at least one and perhaps several more of them. Every dollar raised for Nkosi's Haven, including a great many donations that came in following my first ABC News story about her and Nkosi, was accounted for, to the penny. Among the directors on the board of Nkosi's Haven were two well-known Johannesburg businessmen, Gary Scallon and Gary Roscoe, as well as Justice Edwin Cameron, a highly respected member of South Africa's Constitutional Court who was HIV-positive, and with their endorsement and imprimatur, questions about Gail's integrity soon disappeared.

The invitations kept coming, and once again, against her better judgment, Gail asked Nkosi if he would like to go on another trip to the United States, this time to San Francisco and Atlanta and then to Disney World.

He asked whether, if they agreed to go, it would mean she would be able to raise more money for Nkosi's Haven and to purchase a twelve-acre farm outside Johannesburg as the second step in her plans for expansion. When she told him she thought it would be quite helpful but not absolutely necessary, he said, "I would like to be helpful. Let's go."

As they made plans for the trip, the controversy was still raging over not only President Mbeki's views on the cause of AIDS but also his quick and early departure from the AIDS conference, thereby missing Nkosi's speech and his call for the government to approve AZT. It was seen by many as Mbeki's attempt to avoid being upstaged by Nkosi and interpreted by many more as an insult to the boy himself and collectively to the entire AIDS community.

I had stopped by to see Nkosi once more, soon after the conference, just prior to my departure for London. He was clearly quite miffed with the president of his country. He had taken it personally. "In Durban, I saw Thabo Mbeki sitting one chair away from me, and his wife was sitting next to me," he told me, "and he didn't say anything to me. His wife was very nice, and she talked to me a lot and smiled at me and shook my hand, but Thabo Mbeki did not say anything to me. I was really angry with him. Thabo Mbeki did not break the silence on AIDS. Also, I thought his speech was very boring."

Among those who were publicly chastising the president was Dr. James McIntyre, a medical professor and the director of the Prenatal HIV Research Unit at a hospital in Soweto, the largest in South Africa. Regarded as one of the country's most knowledgeable physicians on the subject, McIntyre told me he could sense Mbeki and his team gearing up to take on Nkosi and all AIDS activists in South Africa.

"The government," he said, "has really been challenged by the fact that a mere child has stood up to them and said things they haven't really enjoyed hearing. It's made them have to respond to it—and it's much more difficult to dismiss the real words of a little boy dying of AIDS than to dismiss some ordinary medical researcher like me."

There was some speculation that perhaps the questions brought up in the media about the money Gail was raising for the shelter had been prompted and planted by the government, and Gail was even concerned that, after she had accepted the latest invitation to visit America, the authorities would not allow her to leave South Africa. But nothing happened.

In September she and Nkosi again made the grueling transatlantic trip to New York and then across the country to San Francisco for several fund raising events, all of which were quite successful.

"Everywhere we went, people fell in love with him," Gail said. He gave much the same speech he had delivered at the AIDS conference, and many of those who heard him seemed moved, not only by the words he spoke but by the courage they saw in him, in the stark contrast between a seriously ill little boy and the mature but passionate ideas he so forcefully expressed. "And I must say that many of the people who were impressed with him," Gail said, "also wanted to make contributions to Nkosi's Haven. I think they must have realized that even if he would not be around for much longer, he deserved a monument for what he was willing to do for the mothers and children back home."

Nkosi enjoyed touring the Napa Valley wine country and seeing the Golden Gate Bridge and Fisherman's Wharf and all the usual tourist attractions of Northern California, including, out in the bay, Alcatraz—or, as Gail called the old federal prison, "the Robben Island of America." The highlight of his

trip to the West Coast, however, was an unforgettable lunch
with the comic and actor Robin Williams.

"He is the funniest man, I think, in all the world," Nkosi recalled. "He made me laugh a lot. He made me laugh until
sometimes my body was hurting. He made me laugh so much
I spit out my water once. Maybe twice. I was laughing very
much at Robin. I think he liked me. I think Robin is my
friend."

In Atlanta in mid-September, he and Gail were featured
guests at an international AIDS conference that focused on the
impact of the disease among minority groups—and then on
down to Disney World, where what might have been an exhil-
arating experience for most boys his age was simply one more
exercise in endurance for him. When it was over, he seemed
relieved to be on the plane, headed back home to Africa. Once
again he slept almost the entire trip.

I returned to Johannesburg in December and drove straight
to Gail's house. I could not believe what I saw when Nkosi
answered the bell, could not comprehend how it was possible
for his weight to have dropped so drastically in just the four
months since I'd last seen him. He had become a wisp. His
eyes were sunken, he had lost even more hair, and just taking a
few steps back to the couch seemed to exhaust him.

After a hug I asked the usual small-talk questions about
how he was feeling and what he was doing and was Gail treating him right and when would she be home and how about
Nikki and what was going on with *The Young and the Restless*.

He answered them all in a voice even softer and weaker than I remembered.

He showed me a picture of him and Danny Glover, the actor and AIDS activist who had visited Nkosi's Haven the month before and who, I later learned, had left in tears. Then, during a brief lull in our conversation, he bluntly told me what I think he had been wanting to tell me since I had walked in the door.

"I have an announcement," he said.

"Whoa, stop the presses, buddy," I said.

"And I hope you won't be angry with me."

"Of course I won't be angry with you. I would never be angry with you. Why would I be angry with you?"

"I have stopped taking my medicine," he said.

"Well," I said, not really knowing what to say. "Why would you want to do that?"

"Because it was not helping me," he said. "I know it was not helping me at all, and it was making me feel so bad every day, and it was making me have more diarrhea than I ever had before—and you know how I just hate the diarrhea. I soil my bed, and I soil my clothes, and I try not to, but I can't help it."

I still didn't know what to say to him, although I knew what I wanted to say. I wanted to tell him he was probably right, that it probably wasn't worth it to make himself so miserable, day after day—but I wasn't certain what Gail's view on the subject was, whether she had agreed or whether she was urging him to continue taking his medications. I wasn't even sure he actually had stopped or was simply planning to stop or wanting to stop and was using me as a shield before he broached the subject with her.

When she arrived a few minutes later, frazzled as usual, the first thing he told her was that he had told me.

"Yes, my darling," she said, "and what did Jim say about that?"

"He didn't say anything," Nkosi answered. "He just asked me why, and I told him."

"So what's that all about?" I asked her when we had retreated to the kitchen for a cup of tea.

"It was very hard," she said, "but I had to face facts, however ugly they are. I have always allowed him to make his own decisions about his body. He knows better than anyone else, including his doctors, what is happening inside of him. He knows whether he is feeling better or not—and according to him, the medications weren't helping him. When he ran out, I said I'd get him some more, and he said, 'Mom, I don't want any more,' and I said, 'Are you sure?' and he said yes."

I asked about his CD4 count.

"It can't go any lower," she said.

So I asked the question I had never asked: "How long?"

"Not long," she replied. Tears welled up in her eyes. I reached across the table and touched my cup to hers.

"To however long it is," I said.

The next day Bentson and the crew set up the cameras and lights again at the shelter, whose population had decreased since our last visit: seven mothers, their eleven children, and five other babies whose mothers had died in the months since we'd been there.

Once again Nkosi and I sat knee to knee in the bright tele-vision lights that flooded one of the children's bedrooms. It was crowded with bunk beds and was where he liked to sleep when he stayed overnight. I asked him what Gail had said when he stopped taking his medicines.

He was coughing constantly, and it took a moment for him to find the breath to answer.

"She said it is my . . . she said, I can choose," he said. "'If you want to stop it, stop it.' So, I said, 'Mom, I am stopping.'"

Since Christmas was only a few days away, I inquired about his personal gift list.

"A Dodge Viper," he said. Once more the grin.

"I want a Porsche," I said. "Good luck to both of us."

He knew that I knew he was pulling my leg.

"I actually dream this Christmas of getting all the money we need for our big dream house," he said.

He was referring to the farm outside Johannesburg that Gail had been eyeing for some time, a much larger version of Nkosi's Haven, with enough space for a hundred mothers and children—and, until then, beyond her financial reach.

"We are full here," he continued. "This is a small house, and we hardly have room for anybody else—and that is not fair to all the other mothers and children who are HIV. They are dying, and they have no place to go. They have no place to bring their children and live."

A wonderful wish, I said. "But what do you want for your-self?"

"I haven't thought about it," he said. "Right now I'm just thinking about all the other mothers out there."

At last I found the nerve to ask about his spirit, his grit I had avoided the subject until then because . . . well, because it did not seem to be a question that a boy ought to have to answer. Still, I was certain that if I didn't ask it that afternoon, it would remain unasked forever.

"You're a very sick boy, and things don't look good for you," I said, "yet you still have that great smile and so much courage. Do you understand that you are brave? Do you understand what courage is? Where did you learn to be so brave?"

And Nkosi said, "Well, I don't really think I'm brave. No, I don't believe I am brave."

A lot of people think you're brave, I told him.

"No, I don't think so," he said. "I just never give up. I never give up because I must fight this bad disease I have. Actually, in 1998 I thought I was going to die then, but I said, 'I am not going to give up. I have a lot of work to do for the other mothers and children out there.' And I'm still not going to give up, because there is still a lot of work to do."

That struck me as a pretty damned good definition of courage.

That night we went to a holiday concert at a local school. He took the stage as the only celebrity there and wished everyone a merry Christmas. Even with the microphone at his lips, I could hardly hear him. The next morning, along with some of the older kids from Nkosi's Haven, we drove out into the Johannesburg suburbs to the sprawling training facility of the Kaizer Chiefs, his favorite soccer club. Several of the players interrupted their workouts to spend a bit of time with him and the other children, and they all left with autographs and yellow jerseys. Most of them had them on before they got back to the van, but Nkosi's fatigue was so deep he seemed to lack the energy required to pull it over his head and shoulders. In fact, it occurred to me that perhaps I should carry him back to the parking lot, and I asked him if he wanted to ride on my shoulders.

"No thanks, Jim," he said. "If you carry me, all the other kids will want to ride, too, and I think you're too old for that. I don't want to make you tired."

"How old do you think I am?" I asked.

"Pretty old," he chuckled.

It was the first smile I'd seen on him that day. It was worth the insult.

That afternoon we went to a local mall with Nkosi and Gail to buy presents for the children at the shelter.

"Put him in there," Gail said, pointing to a shopping cart.

"In there?" I said.

"Yeah," she said. "He fits nicely."

And so I lifted a nearly twelve-year-old boy into the cart's baby seat. Facing Gail, riding backward, with his feet protruding through the spaces, he did fit very nicely.

When the shopping was finished and the cart was full, it was time for us to leave—and one by one—James Mitchell, the cameraman, Royden Astrop, the audio engineer, and Clark Bentson, my three longtime friends and colleagues—stepped forward to say good-bye to the boy and to Gail.

When it was my time, I made it as quick and painless for myself as possible. I gave Gail a kiss on the cheek and a rough hug, then turned to Nkosi. But I could not bear to embrace him again. I actually thought he might be injured by my arms.

Instead I touched his cheek with the tips of my fingers and kissed his forehead and gave him mock-strict instructions about his behavior and his responsibility for seeing to it that Gail also behaved herself. When we shook hands, his completely disappeared inside mine. There was no smile.

O n a Friday afternoon a week or so later, just after New Year's Day, Nkosi badgered Gail to let him spend the first weekend of 2001 at the shelter. She feigned opposition to the idea, but with Nikki out on a date that night, she actually thought it might be a good opportunity to indulge herself, to take a nice long bath, curl up with a book and a glass of wine, and just relax. She finally told him he could go, helped him pack a few clothes in a backpack, and drove him to the house. At the curb she leaned over and kissed him, opened the car door, then handed him his backpack.

"And 'Kosi," she said.

He turned.

"Be a gentleman."

He smiled. "Right, Mom. Always a gentleman."

He had some money stashed away that someone had given him, and he showed it to Grace, the matron of the shelter, and asked if he could treat the kids to some pizza that night. She told him that since dinner was nearly on the table, perhaps the pizza would be a better idea on Saturday night. He made a face but quickly agreed and sat down to another of his favorite meals: roast chicken with potatoes, rice, and gravy. Afterward he asked if he could take a bath.

Grace filled the tub, helped him undress, assisted him over the side, and watched him slide his tiny body into the steaming water.

"That too hot?" she asked.

He smiled.

She left him for a few minutes and returned to find him still soaking, eyes closed, blissfully relaxed. She asked if he wanted to be washed, and, opening his eyes, he said not yet.

As Grace was leaving the bathroom once again, out of the corner of her eye she saw his body stiffen, saw it racked by a quick series of violent spasms, and saw his eyes roll back into his head.

She called his name, but he did not respond.

She screamed for help and lifted him out of the water. Even as small as he was, it was no easy task because of the spasms. The other mothers carried him to the bedroom where he liked to sleep while Grace called Gail. She drove "like Michael Schumacher," she said, from her house to the shelter, helped load him into the rear seat—he was still naked but swathed in blankets and towels and lying across Grace's lap—then sped to the nearest hospital, using her cell phone on the way to alert his doctors, who informed the emergency room of his imminent arrival.

Everyone tried to do something—anything—but there was nothing to be done.

The seizure had caused massive brain damage. From the moment it had begun, Nkosi had immediately descended into a comatose state, eyes closed, breathing labored, unable to speak, to know, to respond, to smile.

In a day or so, when it was clear that nothing else could be done for him at the hospital, he was transferred by ambulance to the house where he had spent the last nine years of his life, carried into the bedroom with all his stuffed animals and posters and photographs with presidents and famous actors, and laid on the soft, clean bed where he had slept for three thousand nights.

It was the consensus of his doctors that he would soon die, and his seizure and impending death were big news in South Africa.

AIDS BOY STRICKEN, one tabloid headline read.

Another said AIDS BOY NEAR DEATH.

In London a clerk in the ABC Bureau had brought me an overnight wire-service story with the details of his condition. I was on a plane to Johannesburg late that night.

When I arrived at the house the next afternoon, it was besieged by reporters and correspondents, camera crews and photographers. The street was filled with television vans, microwave trucks, and crowds of South Africans either curious or simply wishing to express their grief. Inside, it was only slightly calmer. Telephones were ringing, pots and pans were rattling in the kitchen, meals and drinks were being served to friends who had come to help—and Gail, looking as gaunt as one of the women who had come to live in Nkosi's Haven, was trying to make some sense of what had happened to the boy.

She couldn't, of course—other than accepting the lethal logic of AIDS.

His principal physician, Dr. Ashraf Coovadia, would say much the same thing to me. "It's sad and it's tragic, but unfortunately it's a daily event for South African pediatricians like me. I certainly didn't opt for pediatrics to see children die, but it's just very commonplace now. It's a daily event. The disease and the virus are marching on."

The only medical alternative that remained for Nkosi, he said, was the application of palliative therapy, "not to make him well but just to keep him comfortable and free from pain." Dr. Coovadia is a quiet man, a man of great dignity and enormous compassion for the scores of infected infants and children he treats. He could never bring himself to speak to Nkosi or any of them about their inevitable fates. "It is just so abnormal," he said, "so beyond what we all have come to see as the natural cycles of life, to have so many hundreds of children dying."

That afternoon Gail and I retreated to the patio beside the pool.

"I can't understand why his little heart is still beating," she said.

I said I thought it was the heart of a warrior.

"Yeah," she agreed, "but even the bravest warrior knows when the battle is over."

I asked her what she had learned from her years with the boy.

"I think," she said, "the lesson for me is acceptance. Unconditional acceptance. He has accepted us totally, and through that he has taught me unconditional love and unconditional acceptance—and that's what I'd like for the rest of South Africa to learn. You can love and accept and care for infected people and not discard them like so much rubbish in the trash bin.

"I believe in giving and receiving. One won't necessarily receive from the same people one gives to, but there is an invoice for everything one does. It's the isolation of trauma that's more damaging than trauma itself. I know how that feels—so, in the end, this giving is a kind of receiving."

We stared in silence at the water shimmering in the summer sun.

"I'd love for him to talk to me just one more time," she sighed, "because I don't know if there is some unfinished business for my little guy and that's why he's lingering. That's why he's hanging on."

After a moment she said, "I don't want him to be afraid of dying, Jim, and I don't want him to die. I just don't want him to be afraid of it, I really don't. I don't know. Maybe he just doesn't want to go yet. I do know this: I do know he doesn't want to be like this. I mean, be the way he is."

She asked if I had seen him. When I said I had not, she said, "Maybe you'd better not."

Several nurses had been hired to look after him, and a steady stream of visitors came to the bedroom door, stopped for a look, and left. Among the visitors over the next few days were Mrs. Mbeki and Winnie Madikizela-Mandela, Nelson Mandela's ex-wife. They stayed for an hour or so, quietly discussing Nkosi's condition and prognosis with Gail, complimenting her for her care of him and her pioneering work at the shelter, had a cup of tea, and left in a crush of media.

His grandmother, Ruth, and his sister, Mbali, also arrived and spent an entire day at the house. Inside, the grandmother and Gail quietly and calmly discussed plans for Nkosi's funeral. Outside, questioned by reporters, Ruth had nothing but kind words for Gail and for her treatment of her grandson.

Mbeki's chief of staff, Frank Chikane, also stopped by to pay his respects, but the president never appeared.

Friends came to take turns sitting with Nkosi. One afternoon Nikki—by then twenty years old—sat holding his hand, whispering into his ear. "Tomorrow, 'Kosi," she told him, "we'll sit in the garden, you and I, and we'll watch the birds."

Rather unconvincingly, she later told me she thought he had squeezed her hand.

Eric Nichols, the boy who had become Nkosi's first friend at Melpark Primary, stopped by often to see his old classmate, to spend a few moments at his bedside.

Nkosi's condition was unchanging from day to day. Never any better, never any worse. The media vigil continued on the sidewalk and in the street outside the gates of the house.

Gail came to let me in one morning and asked urgently for a cigarette. "I need a twelve-volter," she said.

That afternoon she said, "I looked at his body the other day, and I said that if I had such a body I would sue. I don't want him ever to see the way he looks now. That thin, emaciated face. My God. You know, before his seizure, before he became bedridden, he had to hold tight onto his pants to keep them from falling off, even while he was wearing a belt—and I would look at him and think to myself, 'Dear heavens, my baby, my baby, my darling.'"

On the afternoon of my flight back to London, I stopped to say good-bye again. In my previous time at the house, I had been reluctant to see Nkosi except from a distance, from down the hall through the open door to his bedroom. This time I went in. A feeding tube protruded from his nose. He had eaten no solid food since his last meal—the roast chicken—at the shelter. I had tried to steel myself against what I'd assumed would be his appearance—but nothing, I think, could have prepared me for what had happened to him.

He was lying beneath a blanket, with both arms exposed. Even through the long sleeves of his pajamas, the outline of his bones was visible. There was no more flesh to hide them. I was looking at a skeleton. Under the blanket there was almost nothing to suggest the presence of a human body of any size. Just a small mound, no larger than one of his stuffed animals.

Suddenly it struck me that, little by little, Nkosi was simply disappearing, that one day soon Gail would come into the bedroom to say good morning and discover that her darling boy had simply vanished.

I nodded to the nurse seated on a stool by the bed, walked to the other side, and stretched myself out next to him. Although he was alive, there was no visible sign of it, no movement of respiration from the small lump beneath the covers. I touched his hand—it seemed to me to be the hand of a newborn baby—then wrapped it in mine. There was not the slightest indication of a pulse.

I propped my head on an elbow and watched him for a while, then released his hand and lay flat for a few moments staring at the ceiling, remembering the boy he had been— the boy with the giggles, the boy with all the laughter, the mischievous boy with the light in his eyes, the boy with that marvelous, magnificent grin—and in those moments of remembering, with that boy on the screen of my mind, I found at least a small shred of comfort.

I raised myself, leaned across, and kissed his forehead.

"So long, champ," I said.

At the door I turned for what I knew was one last look.

Somehow I managed not to cry until I was on the plane that night.

For five more months, he somehow kept a feeble hold on life. In early February his twelfth birthday was celebrated by his former classmates at Melpark Primary—there were songs, a cake and ice cream, and several prayers were said for him. A few days later, after another particularly severe seizure, he reentered the hospital. After a brief stay, during which he was stabilized, he was brought back home to his bed.

To prevent sores from developing, the nurse turned his body every two hours. Several times daily the tranquilizer Valium was added to his intravenous feeding to reduce the incidence of the seizures. But there was no hope of recovery; there was only the question of how much longer he could last.

The crowd standing vigil outside the Johnson house gradually diminished over the weeks, but it never completely disappeared. It included its share of wild-eyed eccentrics and religious fanatics who believed they could cure the dying boy. One man severely cut himself to expose a rib he wished to present to Nkosi as a means of healing. He was quickly taken away by police but returned the next night and tried to gain entry to the house by scaling the wall. He was thwarted again.

Gail was receiving hundreds of letters every day. One local woman wrote that Nkosi was in fact an angel dispatched from paradise to earth to teach human beings the lessons of love and courage. Gail, who had not lost her sense of humor despite the stress and pressure of those long and painful weeks, laughed when she read that particular note. "Clearly this woman has never met Nkosi," she said. "Anyone who has ever dealt with my darling boy would know for sure that he is definitely *not* an angel and never was."

Those familiar with Zulu traditions explained Nkosi's survival as a waiting period. He could not die, they said, until his father had performed a Zulu ritual in which ancestral spirits were informed of the boy's virtues so that he could be accepted by them as a part of the family. But no father of Nkosi's stepped forward. Gail was sensitive to such lore and allowed an ancient cleansing ceremony called *ukugezwa,* involving washing the body with goat's bile, to be performed on Nkosi.

On the last day of May, a daily South African newspaper, the *Sowetan,* which in the past I had always found to be respectable, published an off-the-wall story about the claims of a woman named Hilda Khoza. A former laboratory technician, she now described herself as a "reflexologist," and although she had never actually met either Gail or Nkosi, she had spent some time, she said, with Ruth, the boy's grandmother. Nkosi should not be in a coma, the woman told the author of the article; he should be in school. His only problem was constipation, not AIDS, she said, and she was certain Nkosi was the victim of abuse by Gail. She described HIV as a man-made virus created by white scientists whose only motivation was personal profit and racial genocide, and she boasted of having successfully treated some of South Africa's most prominent politicians living with HIV or AIDS. She also claimed to have cured breast cancer and warned women against taking birth-control pills.

The story was yet one more sad exploitation of the long tragedy of Nkosi's life, and yet when someone brought it to Gail's attention, she could only laugh. She said she thought most everyone would see the woman as patently a fraud. The one certain fact about Nkosi's condition, she said, was that he was definitely *not* constipated.

The papers on that last day of May also included reports of an appearance in the Parliament by the South African minister of health, Manto Tshabalala-Msimang, in which she announced that the government had no plans to make antiretroviral drugs available and reiterated for what seemed the hundredth time her view that AZT does not cure AIDS.

In the early hours of the following morning, Gail abruptly awoke in her bedroom. She sensed that Nkosi needed or wanted her presence beside him. Moving carefully in the silent predawn darkness, she tiptoed down the hall to his room. The nurse was dozing. Gail sat down beside Nkosi, took his hand, and spoke softly to him, talked to him about all their good times, about the children at the shelter and how much they missed him, about the cards they had made for him, about the plans for a new shelter, their big dream house with so much space for so many mothers and their children, about the dog and the cats, about almost everything they had shared in their lives together.

At twenty minutes to six, as the sun began to rise on South Africa, Xolani Nkosi Johnson died. He weighed about twenty pounds.

It was a Friday, the first day of June—twenty years to the day since the first case of AIDS was officially recognized for what it was.

Gail leaned over and kissed him. "I love you," she whispered. "Go quietly, my darling boy."

E verything was ready and had been for quite some time. Gail and Ruth Khumalo had begun discussing funeral plans soon after Nkosi's first seizure in early January. In late April, during the last visit by his grandmother and sister, those plans had been finalized. A plot had been chosen and purchased in the sprawling West Park Cemetery. A white casket had been purchased by friends, and a prominent tailor in Durban had fashioned a fine white burial suit.

The house on Third Street was quietly busy, as friends and AIDS activists gathered to provide comfort, to answer the constantly ringing telephone, and to handle the swarms of reporters gathered outside who clamored for an appearance by Gail, asking for details of Nkosi's last days and his final moments, wanting the schedule for his funeral, straining for information for their stories.

Gail, who had always been most amenable to the media, had come to the gates on Saturday morning. Her appearance was haggard, the grief in her voice unmistakable. She was exhausted and emotionally drained. "I am sad," she said, "but his race was run. I'm proud of my son. He has done more for AIDS in Africa than anyone else, but it's his turn to rest now." After she answered a few questions, she was led gently back into the house.

Reporters found Eric Nichols, Nkosi's friend from school. "I'm glad God has taken him at last," the boy said. "Now he's a loving angel in heaven. I feel empty without him. I miss his smile. He taught me so many things, like not to be frightened, to be strong, and to care for others."

The Sunday newspapers reported that the South African Parliament had unanimously passed a resolution expressing its regret and its condolences, and announced that services for Nkosi would be conducted on Wednesday morning in St. George's Cathedral in downtown Johannesburg. All seemed to be moving as swiftly and as smoothly as could be expected— until the Monday papers appeared, carrying stories about Nkosi's grandmother's objections to the plans. Ruth had not been consulted regarding either the funeral or the place of interment, she said. When her grandson was alive, "he was in jail at the house of that white woman," and now that he was dead, his body was being stolen from his biological family. "That white woman is not his family," she said. "We are his family. He belongs to us now." Moreover, Ruth resurrected the previously discredited allegations that Gail had simply been using Nkosi for personal profit.

That Monday afternoon a local television reporter sat down with Gail, who had agreed to the interview in an effort to calm the rising furor. It didn't help. The reporter, a white woman, said, "There are some who say you cared for Nkosi so

that you could make money out of him." Once again Gail replied that her bank accounts and the records of the shelter
were open and available for the world to see.

By Monday night Ruth and her children—principally Dudu
Gabuza, Cynthia's half sister—along with several neighbors
who had rushed to her side, had hired a hearse from a local funeral home to take Nkosi's body from the mortuary in Johannesburg back to the settlement for services and burial there.
The mortician refused to release it without Gail's permission.
Noisy arguments ensued. Protests and demonstrations were
threatened.

Negotiations were begun between Gail and Ruth's family,
with representatives of the South African Council of Churches
serving as mediators. As the rancorous talks dragged on into
Tuesday evening, the original date and time of the funeral had
to be canceled. Finally, on Wednesday afternoon, the impasse
was broken and a schedule acceptable to everyone announced,
but by then the cathedral was no longer available and alternate
plans had to be cobbled together.

Throughout the struggle Gail tried to remain in the background and had allowed friends and members of the Nkosi's
Haven board to speak for her, but she was adamant about a funeral and burial in Johannesburg. "That was our agreement a
long time ago," she insisted, "and that's what it will be." And it
was—with a few minor modifications.

On Friday morning the cathedral was the scene of a me-
morial service organized by the city's most prominant AIDS
activists, primarily the Treatment Action Campaign, whose
leader, Zackie Achmat, was a fearlessly outspoken critic of

the government's AIDS policies. About five hundred people marched to the cathedral, stopping downtown traffic on the way. Inside, they heard Dean Rowan Smith describe Nkosi as a "brave warrior" who had given "a human face to HIV/AIDS." Smith, no wallflower, also took aim at the health minister's statements in Parliament about the inefficacy of AZT. They came very close, he said, to the infamously callous words of the apartheid era's justice minister, Jimmy Kruger, who had said publicly that the death of Steve Biko had left him cold. "To those thousands who have been using the drug," the clergyman said of the AZT comments, "that must have been a blow deep down in the stomach."

That afternoon Nkosi's body was driven in a hearse to Daveyton, with a police escort from the mortuary in Johannesburg to Victor Ndlazilwane Hall, where a large crowd of black South Africans were waiting to honor the boy. From the hall his body was taken to Ruth's tiny house in the settlement at the edge of the township. Women dressed in white holding lighted candles stood along the route.

At his grandmother's home, the casket was opened, and all through the night hundreds passed by to pay their respects to him and to his aunts and uncles, to his grandmother and to Mbali, his sister. Many who saw the boy in the casket dressed all in white could not believe he was twelve years old.

On a damp and dreary Saturday morning, the hearse retraced its route from Ruth Khumalo's house back to Daveyton, then past the busy airport and on into Johannesburg, to the massive Central Methodist Church, for Nkosi's formal funeral.

The church was jammed with two thousand people, all of whom passed by a poster taped to a stained-glass window in the narthex. Beneath a photograph of a smiling Nkosi was this admonition: "Let the love and courage of Xolani Nkosi Johnson fill your heart with determination to care for the infected and forgotten children of our land." Among the mourners was Kenneth Kaunda, the former president of Zambia, whose own son had died of AIDS. At the front of the church were dozens of wreaths and bouquets, including one from Nelson Mandela and another from the Kaizer Chiefs.

Near the altar, a few feet away from the flower-draped coffin, sat Gail and Nikki, and beside them Mbali and Ruth, who seemed to have turned another corner in her ever-changing views on Gail. To the congregation Ruth said, "Today is the end of Nkosi's journey, but I want to humbly thank the white lady, Gail Johnson, who was led by God."

Just behind the family was a group of mothers and children from Nkosi's Haven, many of whom joined in hymns sung in Zulu, Xhosa, and English before various clergymen rose in their colorful vestments to address the packed sanctuary.

"We must not forget that he was but a child," said the Reverend Brian Oosthuizen, the pastor of Central Methodist. "Yet, because of his disease, he was a man."

The presiding Methodist bishop of Southern Africa, Mvume Dandala, had similar words about Nkosi but was much less gentle with Thabo Mbeki and his government. "Show this country, show these children, some compassion!" he roared from the pulpit to thunderous applause.

The president was absent, which surprised no one. In his

place was Bongani Khumalo, a senior aide to Vice President Jacob Zuma. Khumalo did not speak during the service but had a quote ready for reporters before he entered the church. "Nkosi lived only a dozen years," he said, "but his influence is infinite."

The most poignant moment in the service came when Mbali, by then sixteen years old, stood and spoke. Slowly, haltingly, she read the words she had penned in the previous few days.

> To the only brother I had.
> The only family I had.
> You were a hero to others,
> A young brother to me.
> Poverty separated us.
> Rich side had you.
> Poor side had me.
> But we were together.
> The family bond had us.
> I love you, brother.
> Give my love to Mama
> I miss you both.
> Now I'm stuck with your memory.
> I will miss you,
> Now and always,
> As I am lonely in this world.

The funeral concluded with a song Nkosi had loved to sing, "I Believe I Can Fly," and another written for him, called "Rainbow Child."

The procession wound its way through downtown Johannesburg and out toward the suburbs, arriving at the cemetery just before one o'clock. A sizable crowd had gathered beside the waiting grave. Gail and Nikki huddled together, Ruth and Mbali beside them, and just behind them the mothers and children from the shelter, all standing silently around the tiny white casket as the booming voice of the bishop echoed across the sprawling green hills covered with tombstones, first reading briefly from the Gospels, then offering a formal prayer—and closing with this Shakespearean benediction:

Good night, sweet prince, / And flights of angels sing thee
   to thy rest!

EPILOGUE

A year later I went back to Johannesburg, back to West Park Cemetery, where thick slabs of sod had been laid across Nkosi's grave and new sprigs of grass had taken root around the edges. But the government of Thabo Mbeki was still singing its familiar song, still insisting he had not been wrong about the origins of AIDS, still resisting all efforts—including orders from its own courts—to allow millions of infected South Africans access to the drugs and medicines that would at least enhance their lives, if not save them.

The president was still stubbornly clinging to what he had so often described as "legitimate skepticism" about the "untested" and "dangerous" antiretrovirals, AZT and nevirapine. At one point in the ongoing debate, Mbeki had gone so far as to say that he had never actually met anyone with AIDS.

In fact, in the year since Nkosi's death, as the virus continued to ravage the country, the president's own press secretary,
Parks Mankahlana—whom Mbeki saw nearly every day and
who always sternly admonished reporters *not* to ask questions
about AIDS—died of it. I had not known him well and had
dealt with him only briefly, but he had always struck me as
quite a capable man, a decent warrior in the struggle for a different kind of South Africa, and well aware of the toxic residue
of apartheid; yet his strict allegiance and loyalty to the policies
and pronouncements of Mbeki's government and the African
National Congress had often led him to defend the indefensi-
ble, as when he had suggested that in the long run it would be
better not to provide AZT for infected pregnant women because their unborn children would inevitably become orphans
and "a burden on the state."

After this loyal ANC official's death, the ANC kicked its
propaganda campaign into high gear. The party denied that
AIDS had killed either him or Nkosi. An official party docu-
ment, written by Peter Mokaba—who, like Mbeki, said that
the virus did not exist and no one was dying of AIDS—went
even further. "Parks died," it said, "vanquished by the antiretroviral drugs he was wrongly persuaded to consume. He
died prematurely, but the professionals who fed him the drugs
that killed him remain free to feed others with the same
drugs. They lived to tell us and the world that he died of a
virus they had never found in his body." The same had been
true, Mokaba wrote, for Nkosi. He had been poisoned by his
medication.

The ANC did not go unanswered. Jimmy Carter, the former American president, had traveled to Africa along with Bill Gates Sr., the father of the world's richest man, to drum up support for intelligent and effective AIDS policies. After visiting in a half dozen countries being destroyed by the virus, the pair came to South Africa and sat down with President Mbeki.

Afterward Carter expressed his irritation. "One of the excuses Mbeki makes—which really pisses me off—is that condoms are a Western plot to kill off the African population," Carter said.

Carter also met with Mandela and urged him to intervene with Mbeki. Not long afterward, Mandela did speak publicly on AIDS for the first time. "This is war," he said. "It has killed more people than all previous wars and natural disasters. We must not be debating and arguing when people are dying." Later he was seen wearing a T-shirt on which was printed the words HIV POSITIVE.

Even though by this point the number of HIV infections in South Africa had reached 1,800 per day, more than in any other country in the world, Mbeki did not relent.

For Gail, Mbeki's endless harangues had become so routine as to be almost boring. She instead focused her attention and energies on the tasks she and Nkosi had begun. With increased contributions from South Africans and donors abroad, she purchased not only the house adjacent to Nkosi's Haven but the twelve-acre farm as well and had spent considerable time studying innovative agricultural methods to be applied there. A lot of work remained to make it ready for residents, but she envisioned that once it was, it would be self-sustaining in terms of food and water for the mothers and children who would live there.

Her prominence had not diminished. Over the months since Nkosi's death, she had been honored frequently for her work, including being given the prestigious *South African Jewish Report*'s humanitarian award.

A new library had been added to the original Nkosi's Haven, a gift from one of the many donors who, because of Gail's efforts, had become concerned about infected mothers and their children. And several emergency vehicles—ambulances and CPR vans—were on the streets of Johannesburg bearing Nkosi's name on their doors and hoods. A Japanese foundation had established a fund that would pay the school fees for five of the shelter's children, and other, similar scholarships were in the works.

One afternoon I drove out to visit Nkosi's grandmother, Ruth Khumalo, to ascertain whether she might be helpful if I decided to write at length about her grandson. In the little shack where she had lived for several years by then, we sat facing each other across a rickety old table. At first she seemed amenable to assisting me and pleased that perhaps a book about the boy would result. Then Dudu, one of her daughters, sat down beside me. Instructing her mother to remain silent, Dudu took over the conversation.

"You will be making money from such a book?" she asked.

I said I would hope that it would generate some money and that if it did, most of it would go to Nkosi's Haven.

"And how much will you be giving us?"

I explained that my plan was to assume financial responsibility for Mbali's education—to pay for all costs, including books, lunches, uniforms, transportation, tuition and fees for as long as she remained in school, including college.

Dudu vigorously shook her head. "No, no, no," she said. "I mean, how much money will you be giving us if we talk to you?"

I said I hadn't thought about that and reiterated what I considered to be the virtues of my plan to help with Mbali's education.

"No," Dudu said.

I asked how much money she had in mind.

Without blinking an eye, she said fifty thousand dollars.

"And if I don't give you fifty thousand dollars, you and your family and your mother will not talk to me?"

"That's right," she said.

I thanked Ruth Khumalo for her time and left.

Later that week Gail sat on her bed reading a letter Nkosi had written to her after his first year in school. It was merely a listing of the friends he had made, the books he had read, the things he liked and did not like about Melpark Primary, but she often unfolded it and found in its simple childish scrawl a gathering of comfortable memories.

It had taken her months before she finally willed herself to pack up his clothes. Some would be given to children at the shelter, the rest would be donated to local charities. She had also transferred one of Nkosi's favorite stuffed animals, a large tiger, to her own bedroom.

"I suppose it's rank silliness," she said, "but every day I see it, and it reminds me that my darling boy fought like a tiger— and so, when I see it and remember that, it inspires me for yet another day to go out and try to do the same."

Nkosi's room had hardly changed at all, except that it had a new occupant. A few days after Christmas, the child-welfare authorities had delivered a little boy to 48 Third Street. He was not quite a week old and had been abandoned by his mother on the steps of a local hospital.

Would she take him? Gail was asked.

She gathered him in her arms and into her family. She named him Thabo.

ACKNOWLEDGMENTS

Like almost every other author I know or have read, I am indebted to a number of friends and colleagues for their sustained interest in my effort to tell this story, and, with all the sincere effusiveness that can possibly be expressed in the printed word, I thank them, one and all.

Still, this book had but one single godfather: my longtime pal, rabbi, and brother, David Halberstam. Without his encouragement—indeed, without his *basso profundo* demands that I damned well write it—it would not have been written. For that and for a thousand other kindnesses . . . I thank him.

My other best friend, Patience O'Connor—who also happens to be my wife—played an equally important role in this enterprise. Already accustomed to, though never happy with, my long absences on network assignments, she not only tolerated the further detachment required for writing but lovingly insisted that I devote as much time alone as necessary for its completion. For that, and for countless other gifts, I thank her.

My five daughters—Karen, Kris, Katie, Liz, and Lacie—have always been enthusiastic cheerleaders for my work, and their support and encouragement for this part of it was a grand gift for their father.

Among my television comrades, I am especially indebted to Clark Bentson, a consummate producer and thoroughly compassionate human being who knows this story as well as I and maybe—or maybe not, given his instinct to move on to the next one—could have told it much better.

Similarly, those at ABC News who either encouraged or indulged my passion for AIDS in Africa are to be remembered for their wisdom, their foresight, and their willingness to devote precious minutes of network time to stories that were, in essence, ugly and unpleasant. Paul Friedman, who always managed somehow to be more of a journalist than an executive, is a memorable model for his intelligent interest in and concern for a forgotten place on the planet. I will always be grateful to him for his sense of today's unmistakable tragedy and tomorrow's cloudy promise.

I offer my thanks as well to Scott Moyers, my brilliant young editor, a fellow Southerner and an everlastingly patient fellow who skillfully led me from anecdote to narrative, then presided over the formulation of a finished manuscript with all the nuanced guile of—I can't decide which—a riverboat gambler or an itinerant evangelist. I cannot fail to omit Sophie Fels and Janie Fleming, his indefatigable assistants, in my collection of gratitude, nor can I forget the exemplary work of Maureen